Mental Health Assessment in Occupational Therapy

An Integrative Approach to the Evaluative Process

Edited by
Barbara J Hemphill MS, OTR, FAOTA

SLACK Incorporated, 6900 Grove Road, Thorofare, New Jersey 08086

Printed in the United States of America

Library of Congress Catalog Card Number: 86-42925

ISBN: 1-55642-004-8

Published by: SLACK Incorporated
              6900 Grove Rd.
              Thorofare, NJ 08086

Last digit is print number: 10   9   8   7   6   5   4   3   2   1

CONTENTS

RESEARCH ANALYSIS

APPENDICES

DEDICATION

Dedicated to my mentors and colleagues who supported me, inspired me, encouraged me, and had faith in me.

For the ease of those who read
Mental Health Assessment, male gender pronouns
have been used throughout the book,
unless female gender is specified.
We regret there are no concise or appropriate
unisex terms that could have been used instead;
the invention of these are awaited with impatience.

FOREWORD

In 1978, occupational therapists working in mental health settings identified developing, standardizing, and sharing patient assessments as the second highest critical issues affecting their practice. In the years following that survey, many therapists have attempted to help resolve that problem. No one has had more impact than editor Hemphill and the contributing authors in the first edition of *The Evaluative Process in Psychiatric Occupational Therapy*. This book reviewed established assessments and introduced several newly researched instruments. The wide adoption of this text by faculty members and clinical practitioners helped focus and improve the assessment aspect of psychiatric practice.

This new edition continues the momentum into new territory. It includes two frequently used assessments: the interest checklist and the activities configuration, which were not included in the first edition. This volume also reflects the changing character of psychiatric occupational therapy practice by including information on practical assessments related to daily life situations. The current practice climate demands more tools of this nature. In addition, Hemphill recognizes the resurgence of interest in pre-vocational testing and has included a chapter on this topic.

For occupational therapy students, this book provides descriptive information on the evaluation process and specific evaluation instruments. Practicing therapists will find more evaluations to add to their repertoire.

This book moves our profession closer to achieving the goal of measuring our impact in order to make our therapy more efficient and effective. We can respond with more confidence to the current emphasis on quality assurance, accountability, and cost effectiveness with the availability of resources such as this compilation.

December 1986
Elizabeth A. Moyer, MS, OTR, FAOTA
Tallahassee, Florida

ACKNOWLEDGEMENTS

Tina Barth wishes to acknowledge the contribution of Win Leav, COTA, for her assistance and perseverance in developing the original graphics and color selections, and Sarah A. Deal, MS, OTR, for her assistance with the literature review and for her encouragement.

Carol Leonardelli wishes to thank the American Occupational Therapy Foundation and the University of Wisconsin-Milwaukee Graduate School for financial support of this project. The following have provided invaluable input and support to the author in the development of the MEDLS: Robert Alm, Judith Bloomer, Barbara J. Hemphill, James McPherson, Kenneth Ottenbacher, Diane Shapiro, Franklin Stein, Mary Pat Taugher, Susan Williams, and Sara Zwirlein. Grateful appreciation is extended to Sara Weideman, Mary Jo Theune, Leanne Wilson, Linda Buyan, and Carlynn Higbie, former students at UW-Milwaukee, and to the 73 occupational therapists who reviewed the MEDLS during its development.

Chapter 5 is adapted from an article by Oakley, Kielhofner, Barris, and Reichler (1986), *Occupational Therapy Journal of Research*, 6, 157-170.

PREFACE

This textbook is a continuation of *The Evaluative Process in Psychiatric Occupational Therapy*. It presents assessments primarily in the behavioral and learning area of human function. This completes and broadens information about assessments that was not included in the previous publication.

The purpose of this textbook is to provide the clinician and student with current and accurate information about occupational therapy assessment tools used in mental health, to describe in greater detail a model for selecting assessment tools, and to generate research by comparing and contrasting evaluations developed by occupational therapists. No theory or frame of reference is advocated in this text. The selection of assessments was based on three criteria. The assessments were: 1) developed by an occupational therapist, 2) often referenced in the occupational therapy literature, 3) often reported as being used by occupational therapists.

The author did not impose a criteria based on the assessments' usefulness or research development. The intent is to develop a compilation of assessments used in occupational therapy mental health. In order to select assessments, the therapist must know what is available. However, it is not enough to be knowledgeable about assessments, but to select assessments based on clients' needs and the assessment's ability to measure behaviors.

The integrative approach is a model used to evaluate clients. It is a method that can be employed throughout the occupational therapy process. Starting with the data-gathering process, which includes the interview, medical sources, and evaluation, the clinician/student can use several evaluations that will identify dysfunction in the four areas of human function. This material is intended to present a model for which a client can be assessed holistically.

The first chapter establishes the theoretical premise for using the integrative approach to assess clients. Its relationship to goal writing and research is discussed. Thus, the major theme of this textbook is to provide a framework (integrative approach) and rationale for proceeding from the data-gathering process to the selection of occupational therapy assessments used in mental health.

This textbook is organized into three additional sections:

1) The Interviewing Process. This section is revised to include more in-depth information about the process of interviewing, the

concept of the third ear, and the listening components of interviewing.

2) The Assessments in the Areas of Human Function. This section is divided into two parts. Each part includes assessments that reflect area of human function in the integrative approach. Occupational behavior and learning assessments are described. These assessments were developed and reported on in published and unpublished manuscripts. There are two chapters that deviate from the established criteria. They are: ADL Assessments Used with the Older Adult, and Pre-Vocational Assessments in Mental Health. These chapters were included to give the reader an overview of assessments used in specific settings. At most, they are assessments that were developed by occupational therapists. A few are assessments that occupational therapists frequently use to assess a psychiatric client.

3) Research. The last section is a review of occupational therapy assessments used in mental health. The intent is to compare and contrast these assessments in order to generate further development. In order to accomplish the last section, each writer discusses the theoretical base, the administration, the utilization, and the research of his or her specific assessment. This section is not intended to give judgment about the "good or "bad" of each assessment, but an attempt to give a fair analysis. It is up to the practicing therapist reading this text to decide the value of an assessment tool.

The author hopes that by compiling these assessment tools, therapists learn what is available for assessing clients in the mental health setting. Students are provided with ideas for conducting research and the realization of the potential of assessments. Many of our assessments need further research. Discussing their design and methodology may enhance research in this area.

CONTRIBUTORS

Roann Barris, EdD, OTR, FAOTA

Tina Barth,
MA, OTR, CRC
Clinic Director
Mental Health Services
BRC Human Services Corporation
Private Practice
Health Related Consulting Services
New York, New York

Betty Risteen Hasselkus,
PhD, OTR, FAOTA
Assistant Professor
Occupational Therapy Program
School of Allied Health Professions
Univesity of Wisconsin-Madison

Barbara J. Hemphill,
MS, OTR, FAOTA
Associate Professor
Department of Occupational
Therapy
Western Michigan University
Kalamazoo, Michigan

Alexis D. Henry, MS, OTR/L
Rehabilitation Coordinator
McLean Hospital
Belmout, Massachusetts

Gary Kielhofner,
DrPH, OTR, FAOTA
Associate Professor and Department
Head of Occupational Therapy
College of Associated Health
Professions
University of Illinois at Chicago

Carol A. Leonardelli, MS, OTR
Assistant Professor
Occupational Therapy Program
University of Wisconsin-Milwaukee

Linda Kohlman McGourty,
MOT, OTR
Supervisor of Occupational Therapy
Valley Medical Center
Renton, Washington

Gail Hills Maguire, PhD, OTR
Associate Professor, Graduate
Coordinator
Department of Occupational Therapy
Florida International University
Tamiami Campus
Miami, Florida

Linda Ogden Niemeyer, OTR, CVE
Private Practice/Consultant
Work Tolerance Screening, Work
Hardening
Riverside, California

Frances Oakley, MS, OTR
Coordinator, Clinical Research
Occupational Therapy Service
Department of Rehabilitation
Medicine
National Institutes of Health
Bethesda, Maryland

Cindee Peterson, MA, OTR
Professor, Clinic Coordinator
Occupational Therapy Department
Western Michigan University

Joan C. Rogers, PhD, OTR, FAOTA
Professor of Occupational Therapy
School of Health Related Professions
Assistant Professor of Psychiatry
Geriatric Psychiatry and Behavioral
Neurology Module
Western Psychiatric Institute and
Clinic
School of Medicine
University of Pittsburgh

Carol Shaw, MA, OTR
Private Practice/Consultant
Special Lecturer in in Occupational
and Physical Therapy Program
Columbia University

Franklin Stein, PhD, OTR, FAOTA
Director, Occupational Therapy
Program
Professor, Department of Health
Sciences
University of Wisconsin-Milwaukee

CHAPTER 1

AN INTEGRATIVE APPROACH TO THE USE OF OCCUPATIONAL THERAPY ASSESSMENTS IN MENTAL HEALTH

Barbara J. Hemphill, MS, OTR, FAOTA

In the last several years, a proliferation of occupational therapy assessments in mental health seems to have developed. Because of the increasing number of assessments being reported and published, the difficulty of knowing what is available from which to select increases. The criteria for selection are oftentimes unknown. However, there are several factors that therapists report to use in selecting assessments. Among these factors are: the therapeutic setting, the therapist's expertise, educational experiences, theoretical preferences and client population.

The purpose of this chapter is to describe a structure of selecting assessments based on a theoretical premise that allows therapists to use a variety of assessments to achieve an integrative view of the client with emotional problems. The selection process begins by identifying the client's dysfunction and liabilities in four aspects of human function, which will be described later in the chapter. The next step is to develop intervention and methods of treatment that reflect the four aspects of human function. The chapter will first cover the assumptions about the integrative approach to client assessment. This is followed by a discussion of the areas of human functions. In order to describe a structure for assessment selection, the integrative approach will be detailed by outlining the evaluative process. The chapter will conclude by discussing the criteria for critiquing assessment for use in mental health.

The integrative approach to client assessment has several assumptions. First, that assessments are developed out of a theoretical base. This implies that when the therapist is employing an assessment, he is operating under the theory for which the assessment was developed, and he will then use that theory for intervention. Therefore, the use of one assessment to identify client needs implies that the client has problems only in the area for which the assessment has been made and the client will be treated based on the results of that one assessment.

An example of the danger of using one assessment is expressed in a common question that is asked. "Do you know of an assessment tool for the older population?" The usual answer to this question is "no," because the behaviors being assessed are unknown. There is an assumption in the question that by using the same assessment, all older people in an acute setting need to be assessed for the same behaviors. If treatment goals are based on the same assessment, there is the danger that intervention could be relatively the same for everyone. Since there are individual differences among populations, there is also the possibility that clients' needs that are not assessed by one instrument are overlooked. The question of population is only relative to the norm group for which the assessment has been researched, and this is important to keep in mind. However, there are assessments that are not specific for any age group and should be considered.

The second assumption is that an integrative approach assures that the client is viewed from a holistic philosophy. This means that using the four areas of human function to assess the client encourages the therapist to administer a variety of assessments that are based on different theoretical premises. This may imply an eclectic view. However, this approach does not allow the therapist to pick and choose fragments from various assessments that support his biases and preconceived ideas, but instead enables the therapist to integrate many theories and techniques for the purpose of assessing the client in mental health. An example is a therapist who practices analytical theory and finds it necessary to administer an assessment that evaluates activities of daily living.

By employing the evaluative process, assessment tools are selected based on clients' needs because it is often the case that clients have difficulties in more than one area. Through the data collection and interviewing process, clients' dysfunction and liabilities can be identified. Once this has been accomplished, the appropriate assessments are selected. The emphasis here is that more than one assessment is possible. In addition, it is possible that more than one theoretical premise on which assessments are based can be employed. The appropriate question would be "are there assessment tools for the older person that can evaluate occupational performances and be administered in a short period of time?" This type of question widens the assortment of assessments from which to select, therefore, using more than one assessment. The assumption is that even though the assessments are based on different theoretical premises, the use of one assessment does not imply a rejection of other seemingly divergent assessments.

The theoretical premise that allows therapists to use more than one assessment tool lies in the occupational therapy literature in which authors discuss the integration of seemingly conflicting frames of references. In 1968,[1] it was recognized that educators and therapists needed a system for integrating numerous bodies of knowledge with occupational therapy practice. The first attempt was made by Owen. The author reviewed the Eleanor Clarke Slagle lectures presented in the 1960s to identify the underlying philosophy inherent in occupational therapy. The author concluded that occupational therapy practice related to three schools of thought. They were: realism, existentialism, and pragmatism. This view was seen as tending toward eclecticism.[2]

Later, Dunning supported the existential view. The author stated that existentialism included three simultaneous modes. They were: psychological, social, and biological.[3] These three modes reflect areas of human function. The psychological included the affective aspect of the individual. The social included the influences of the environment on the individual, and the biological included the physical aspects of the individual. These areas of human function also reflect theories about human function. The psychological area relates to the analytical theories, the social area relates to the behavioral theories, and the biological area relates to developmental, biochemical, and neurological theories. Thus, Dunning's modes can be referred to as aspects of human function. They occur simultaneously "because man participates in all three at the same time. There is no hierarchy or priority system among them." This suggests that clients could be approached from the three separate modes or aspects of human function reflected in the treatment plan. The modes are equally important and essential to the occupational therapy process.

In 1970, Mosey published the book *Three Frames of Reference for Mental Health*.[4] The author proposed three frames of reference: the analytical, developmental, and acquisitional. They were intended to be used eclectically. Eclectic means to select from various sources what seems to be best. Mosey did not suggest a structure for which the eclectic approach could be applied to practice. Therefore, my colleagues could not tell me how this could be accomplished, but that they were using more than one frame of reference in their practice.

If these aspects of human function, described by Dunning, were applied to the use of frames of references, then more than one could be utilized with the client. Therefore, it would be appropriate to draw from a variety of assessments that are based on different theoretical premises to determine treatment methods for clients. Mosey states that "in the process of intervention with a client, more than one frame of reference is often used to guide practice.[4] This is particularly true when the individual has multiple problems in areas of dysfunction.[5]

Later, Clark attempted to organize the practice of occupational therapy by categorizing four theoretical approaches. They were: adaptive performance, biodevelopmental, facilitating growth and development, and occupational behavior. The author did not provide a structure for integrating the various approaches that would link practice to theory. However, the author did agree that "no one theory can be expected to guide professional action. Instead, a therapist must knowledgeably select and use those theories appropriate to a specific practice situation."[6] Other authors[7,8] have proposed methods of organizing occupational therapy concepts. However, the authors have not provided a practical means for which to apply conflicting theories which seem to characterize occupational therapy practice.

The selection process begins by identifying the client's dysfunction and liabilities in the aspects of human function. The results gleaned from the assessments lead to the application of various frames of reference. A frame of reference provides directions as to how the practitioner interacts in the intervention process.[5] After the assessment process, the treatment process begins by writing goals that reflect the dysfunction and liabilities in the aspects of human function. Therefore, the therapist is applying the concept of the integrative approach to occupational therapy treatment in mental health.

In summary, the literature demonstrated that more than one theoretical premise can be used to guide practice, if one is to serve clients in the biological, psychological, and sociological aspects of human function. The central theme demonstrated that the eclectic approach is recognized as legitimate for occupational therapy. However, an undisciplined eclectic approach is not a sound rationale for indiscriminate use of concepts and techniques. A more systematic approach to the use of occupational therapy tools and methods is needed. Even though there is a need for a system to integrate occupational therapy knowledge, no structure is identified by which this could be accomplished.

Therefore, an integrated approach to the profession's theoretical premises, assessment tools, and corresponding frames of reference is being suggested. By providing a visible organization that recognizes the aspects of human function described by Dunning, more than one theory, assessment, and their corresponding frames of reference can be utilized in practice. The integrated approach recognizes four areas of human function. The social area, suggested by Dunning, was expanded to include the behavioral and learning theories as separate areas of human function for convenience of understanding. The integrative approach allows the clinician to use more than one assessment for any given client based on the individual's needs in the areas of human function, rather than on population, clinical setting, therapist's personal preference, or other biases. The definition of the integrative approach to the selection of assessments is the process whereby client dysfunction and liabilities are identified by the utilization of various assessments that reflect four areas of human function—psychological, behavioral, learning, and biological.

Areas of Human Function

Psychological

The psychological area of human function is described in the psychoanalytical theories. Occupational therapy theorists such as Azima[9] and Fidler[10] are included in this area. Projective tests such as the Azima and Fidler Batteries, B.H. Battery,[11] Shoemyen Battery,[12] Goodman Battery,[13] and the Magazine Picture Collage[14] are a few assessments that evaluate the intrapsychic. Attributes such as insight, objective relations, body image, and the use of defense mechanisms are a few factors that are gleaned from projective tests. The psychological function "is the ability to process information from past events and information currently available...as to view one's self, others, and one's life situation realistically. The psychological functions are influenced by and derived from the emotional, feeling part of the human experience".[15] The projective tests allow the therapist to assess the psychological area of human function.

Behavioral

The behavioral area of human function is described in the behavioral theory, commonly known as reinforcement, proposed by B.F. Skinner. Our body of knowledge about the behavioral is found in theories proposed by Reilly and recently by Fidler. Other theories that have expanded upon the occupational behavior theory are included in this area of human function.[16,17] Here the occupational therapist is concerned about the role of the environment in the acquisition of maladaptive behaviors. It involves an analysis of the client's environment and the effect it may have on the person's ability to perform in work, play, and daily living. This area also includes the process of social interaction. Social skills such as communication and group interaction are attributes that are evaluated. Assessments such as the Interest Checklist,[18] Occupational Role History,[19] Life Style Performance Profile,[20] Activity Configuration,[21] Adolescent Role Assessment,[22] and the Bay Area Functional

Performance Evaluation[23] are just a few of the evaluations available to use in this area of human function.

Learning

The third area of human function is learning. The educational theorists such as Bloom,[24] and Harlow[25] are included. The teaching-learning process suggested by Mosey[26] utilizes educational theorists in treatment. The learning area is concerned with the skill level performance of the client. There are two factors with which the therapist must be concerned. First is the cognitive function and second is the level of skill development. Functions that are associated with cognition are: attention, memory, orientation, thinking, conceptualization, intellect, and problem solving. Functions that are associated with skill development are: work skill, ADL, leisure, and social skills. The important factor here is that the evaluation involves a task that assimilates the life skill to be performed. A few of the assessments in the learning area of human function are: Kohlman Basic Living Skills Evaluation,[27] Milwaukee Evaluation of Daily Living Skills,[28] Work Capacity Evaluation,[29] and the Paracheck.[30]

Biological

The fourth area to be discussed is the biological area of human function. This refers to the evaluation of neurological, physiological, and anatomical constructs. Theorists such as: Rood, Brunnstrom, Ayres, and Lorna Jean King are utilized. This area includes test procedures which evaluate the physical well-being of the individual. Therapists are most familiar with Lorna Jean King's research about the assessment and treatment of schizophrenic patients using sensory integrative principles.[31] Most recent is the development of the Allen Cognitive Level Test which measures, with the use of leather lacing, a person's functional level. It is particularly useful in measuring cognitive functioning in depressed and demented clients.[32]

The Integrative Approach

The Evaluative Process

Figure 1-1 illustrates the entire procedure that should be implemented for providing patient care. The evaluative process is contained in the following steps:

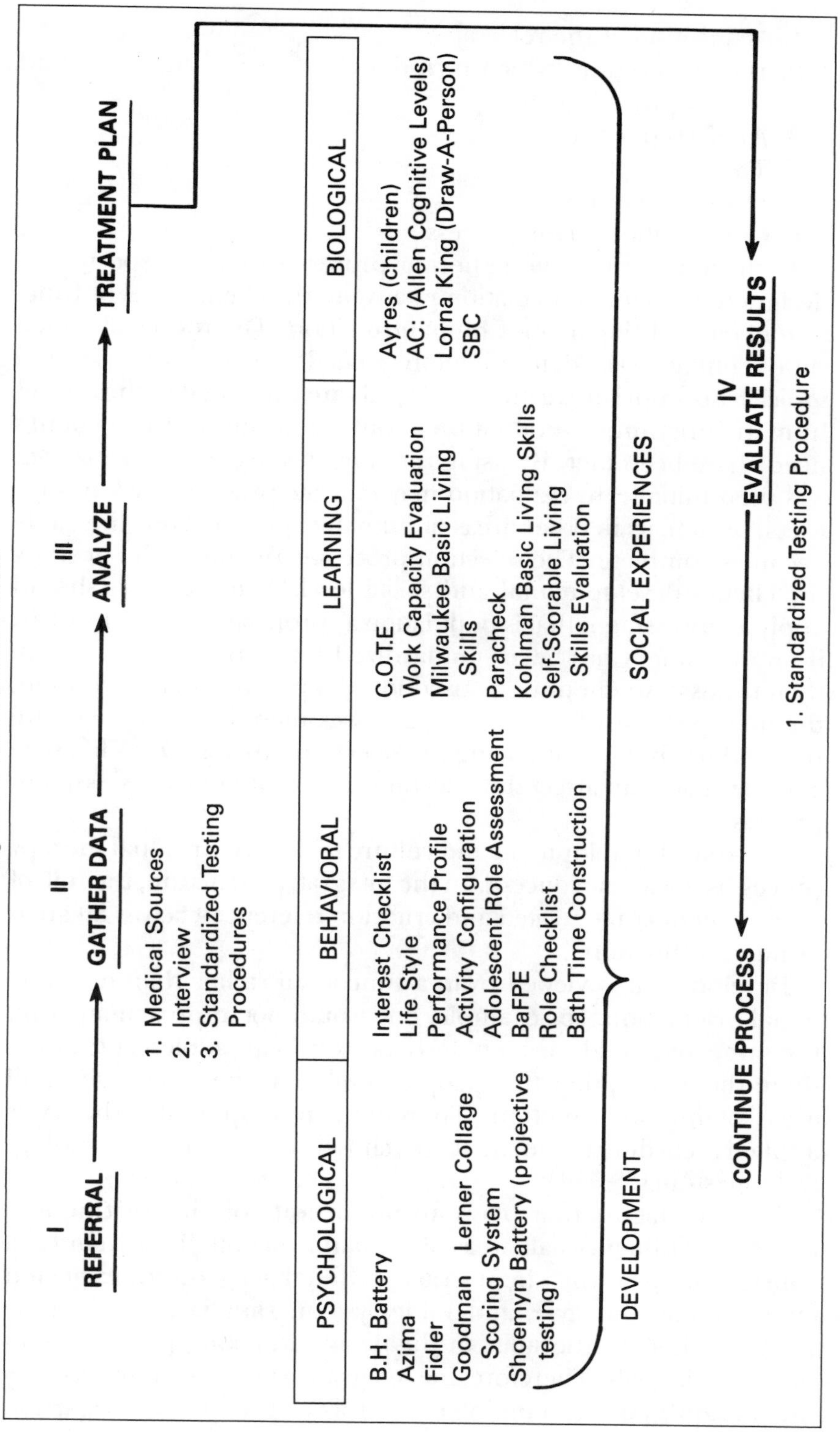

Figure 1-1. The Evaluative Process

I
REFERRAL →

II
GATHER DATA
1. Medical Sources
2. Interview
3. Standardized Testing Procedures

III
ANALYZE → **TREATMENT PLAN**

PSYCHOLOGICAL	BEHAVIORAL	LEARNING	BIOLOGICAL
B.H. Battery	Interest Checklist	C.O.T.E	Ayres (children)
Azima	Life Style	Work Capacity Evaluation	AC: (Allen Cognitive Levels)
Fidler	Performance Profile	Milwaukee Basic Living	Lorna King (Draw-A-Person)
Goodman Lerner Collage	Activity Configuration	Skills	SBC
Scoring System	Adolescent Role Assessment	Paracheck	
Shoemyn Battery (projective	BaFPE	Kohlman Basic Living Skills	
testing)	Role Checklist	Self-Scorable Living	
	Bath Time Construction	Skills Evaluation	

DEVELOPMENT

SOCIAL EXPERIENCES

CONTINUE PROCESS

IV
EVALUATE RESULTS
1. Standardized Testing Procedure

1. Acquisition of the referral
2. Data Collecting (which includes chart review, interview and testing procedures)
3. Analysis of data
4. Treatment plan
5. Evaluation of results
6. Continuation of the process

Each step of the data gathering process should be specifically designed to obtain information relative to the client's level of function in each of the areas of human function. The results obtained should enhance the determination of needs which, in turn, should indicate appropriate treatment. If goals are expressed in the area of human function, re-evaluation should determine if the client's needs have been met. By using the same testing procedure which was used initially, re-evaluation may indicate progress, lack of progress, or deficits in other areas of human function. Thus the circle becomes complete. The selection process is further influenced by the client's developmental and social level. The therapist should apply an assessment that is population appropriate. In other words, if an assessment has been standardized for a specific population, then the assessment must be used for that population. In addition, the therapist must be aware that an assessment is or is not culture free and use judgment during the selection process. One's life style and life space can affect the selection and results of the assessment process.

The role of development and culture in the occupational therapy process is not a new concept. In the integrative structure, the role of development is age related and criterion referenced across all areas of human function.

Development is viewed from a functional rather than dysfunctional orientation. For example, one would not approach an adult the same as a child, or an elderly person as an adolescent; nor is there the assumption that people develop at the same rate in all areas of human function. Therefore, developmental theory is applied according to the client's psychosocial, cognitive, and biological milestones.[32,33,34]

Another factor that plays an important role in treatment is culture. It influences all areas of human function. This includes a consideration of the client's race, ethnic background, expected environment, life style, and value system. Familiarity with these factors assists the therapist in the decision-making process about therapeutic goals. Therefore, the integrative process is enhanced by the therapist's understanding of the role culture plays in regard to experiences and beliefs the client brings to the therapeutic environment.

Figure 1-1 contains all of the necessary components of treatment of our clients. It also contains the assessments that can be selected. They have been categorized according to the four areas of human function.

For a more detailed discussion of the evaluative process, refer to Hemphill, B. (Ed.): *The Evaluative Process in Psychiatric Occupational Therapy,* Thorofare, Slack, Inc., 1982.

Selection Process

The selection process begins by examining the patient's chart. Information should be categorized according to the four areas of human function. The same is true for the interview. Questions should be asked that will provide information about the client's dysfunction and liabilities. By combining this information with information from the chart, one is able to identify the area of human functions that need to be further assessed. This leads to the selection of assessments, and goals are written.

How the therapist can obtain information from an interview that reflects the four areas of human function is illustrated in the following case study (Figure 1-2).

The key in Figure 1-2 indicates which attributes in the case study represent the areas of human function. The psychological area of human function attributes are found in the following description: "appeared depressed, affect was flat, seemed anxious, loneliness and depression, dumb student, and voice indicated anger." The comment about being a dumb student reflects self-esteem. Self-esteem, according to Mosey, is a function of the psychological area.[15] The behavioral area of human function is represented by comments such as "getting along in school," "problems in establishing friendships," and "she and her parents do not get along." The point to remember here is that the therapist is looking at the client's environment and identifying what influence it might be having behaviorally on the client. There are no learning deficits. If there was additional information about the "problems in establishing friendships" that indicates a lack in skill, perhaps this could be a learning deficit. In the biological, the "neck and back pains" could be a biological deficit. However, it could also be psychosomatic. The therapist would have to gather more information to make a determination.

This case study illustrates two factors. First, the integrative approach is a dynamic and flexible structure for gathering data

> Ms. S. was first interviewed February 24, 1986 while in her room. Patient <u>appeared depressed</u>, her <u>affect was flat</u>, and she <u>seemed anxious</u> throughout the interview. She did not volunteer information. The patient reported *neck and back pains*, <u>loneliness and depression.</u> She stated that she sometimes <u>saw and heard things</u>". Ms. S. is 13 years old and in the 7th grade. When asked how she was getting along in school her reply indicated **problems in establishing friendships** and "staying out of trouble with teachers." The patient further reported that her grades were poor because the teachers didn't like her and she was a <u>dumb student anyway</u>. When asked if she used drugs her reply was "no." Ms. S. was asked about her home life. She stated that **she and her parents do not get along**. At this point in the interview the patient appeared more anxious. She shifted in her chair and the tone of her <u>voice indicated anger</u>.
>
> <u>The Azima Battery</u> was administered to evaluate <u>self-concept, level of depression</u>, ***problem solving ability, work tolerance,*** <u>presence of psychosis, level of anger and frustration tolerance</u>. The results show low <u>self-esteem, impulsivity</u>, ***poor work and*** <u>frustration tolerance and extreme anger</u>. ***Problem solving ability*** is normal and evidence of <u>psychosis is absent</u>. Patient's goals are:
>
> 1. <u>improve self-esteem through successful experience with structured activities.</u>
> 2. ***teach interpersonal skill by participation in group activities.***
> 3. ***encourage good work habits.***
> 4. <u>allow expression of anger through constructive structured activities.</u>
> 5. **explore further the relationship between her and her family.**
>
> **Key**
>
> | | |
> |---|---|
> | <u>   </u> | Psychological area of human function |
> | **Bold type** | Behavioral area of human function |
> | ***Bold italic type*** | Learning area of human function |
> | *Italic type* | Biology area of human function |

Figure 1-2. Case study A.

about clients. It utilizes and accommodates various ways of determining client needs. For example, in the case of "problems in establishing friendship" the therapist needs to determine if it is a behavioral or a learning problem. If it is a learning problem and a lack of a skill in establishing friends, then the frame of reference would indicate the teaching-learning approach. If it is a behavioral deficit, it may be merely the lack of opportunity to meet people. Thus, the therapist would need to utilize a different type of intervention.

The second factor that this case illustrates is the danger of using one assessment. The assessment used was the Azima battery. The Azima battery is a projective assessment that evaluates the psychological area of human function. It also evaluates attributes in the learning area, namely "problem solving ability," and "poor work tolerance." The point to be made here is that no one assessment is pure enough to exclusively assess one area of human function; other assessments might have to be utilized. The learning area was not a problem in this case study. There might be a better assessment among the therapist's repertoire that could evaluate these attributes.

The goals in the psychological area of human function are numbers 1 and 4. In the behavioral, the goals are number 5 and in the learning area are numbers 2 and 3.

The next case study illustrates how more than one assessment can be employed (Figure 1-3). Three of four areas of human function are identified in case study B. In this case study, the Activity Configuration, Kohlman Evaluation of Living Skills, and the B.H. Battery were used. They represent the behavioral, learning, and psychological areas of human function respectively.

The goals in the psychological area are numbers 3 and 4. In the behavioral, the goals are numbers 1, 5, and 6, and in the learning area, number 2.

Each of these case studies illustrates the integrative approach to selection of assessment in mental health. Each step of the data gathering process is specifically designed to obtain information relative to the client's level in the areas of human function. The results obtained enhance the determination of needs in the area of human function. The goals are expressed in the area of human function from which the problem was identified. The corresponding frames of reference which guide practice can then be employed. The specific goals dictate the frame of reference to be used; therefore, more than one frame of reference is used in treatment. In case study A, the analytical frame of reference can be used to accomplish goals 1 and 4. The occupational behavior model can be used to accomplish goal 5, and learning can be used to accomplish goals 2 and 3. Therefore, the therapist is able to justify the goals that are written, because he is able to trace back to the assessments that were used. In turn, the therapist is able to base assessment choice on information obtained from the data gathering and interviewing process. Nothing is left to chance and no assumptions are made about the client. If the data gathering process does not identify a problem in one or more areas of human function, a goal for that area is not written.

The writing of goals in each of the areas of human function is a key concept to using the integrative approach. In each of the goals,

> This 23-year-old white female was interviewed in the clinic. Ms. P. appeared *rigid in the chair,* facial expression reserved and non-expressive. The patient stated she felt depressed and had suicidal thoughts. She complained of **not being able to handle arguments with her husband.** Ms. P. **handles her anger by not talking to her husband and leaving the room.** These arguments center around their children and discipline. She considers herself a good housekeeper. Her appearance at the present time indicated *no problems in self-care.*
>
> Ms. P. is a Practical Nurse but *has never worked.* The patient expressed the **desire to do things** outside the home. She state that **in the past she was always busy with hobbies** and various activities. Since her marriage she hasn't been able to do anything. *Her physical well being appears to be within normal limits.*
>
> **The Activity Configuration** was done to evaluate her use of time. It was found that she spends a great deal of time with housework. **She reported not having the time to develop friends to engage in social events.**
> *The Kohlman Evaluation of Living Skills* was given to ascertain the function in self-care, safety and health, money management, transportation and telephone and work/leisure. *All areas scored within normal limits except leisure.* There are *no plans for future employment.*
> The B.H. was administered to evaluate self-concept, presence of psychosis, degree of anger, and problem solving ability. The results show absence of psychosis, and inadequate problem solving ability. She exhibited a low self-concept, and high degree of anger. Ms. P's goals are:
>
> 1. **evaluate her dyadic and group interaction.**
> 2. *teach her problem solving skills.*
> 3. build self-concept through successful activities.
> 4. encourage self-expression (anger) through constructive unstructured activites.
> 5. **explore relationship with husband.**
> 6. **identify and use leisure activities through awareness of community resources.**
>
> **Key**
>
> | | |
> |---|---|
> | _____ | Psychological area of human function |
> | **Bold type** | Behavioral area of human function |
> | ***Bold italic type*** | Learning area of human function |
> | *Italic type* | Biology area of human function |

Figure 1-3. Case study B.

how the goal is expressed identifies the area of human function and the frame of reference that is being used. The analytical frame of reference is expressed in terms such as "encourage self-expression," and "allow expression," and "improve self-esteem." The behavioral frame of reference is expressed in terms such as "identify and use leisure activities" and "explore relationships." The learning frame of reference is expressed in terms such as "teach her." "Teach" is a key term to the learning frame of reference.

Criteria for Selecting Assessments

In order to select among numerous assessments from the areas of human function, there needs to be a criteria. This criteria can be use to determine the usefulness of an assessment. The following questions are guidelines to the selection process. This is discussed further in Chapter XIII.

1. What theoretical premise is the assessment based on? It could be such constructs such as: psychoanalytic, object relations, occupational behavior, occupational choice, skill acquisition, and sensory integration.

2. For what population is the instrument designed? For what setting(s) is the instrument appropriate? This could be a nursing home for the elderly, an adolescent acute care or an institutionalized schizophrenic.

3. What are the behaviors being assessed and are they in measurable terms? How are the behaviors scored? This concerns the measurability of behaviors and how they are scored: Is there a rating scale? Is there meaning to the score?

4. Are there any studies reported regarding validity, reliability, or standardization. These studies can be very valuable in determining if the changes in behavior are measureable. Therefore, one can show an improvement in the client.

5. Is the procedure for administering the instrument clear? How is the instrument administered? Is the protocol standardized? The therapist would want to know if this instrument is administered by interview, observation, or task.

6. What materials are needed? Such concerns as material costs are important. Whether the materials have to be purchased or can be made is also a determination of use.

7. What area of human function is the instrument designed to test? The area of human function is similar to asking on what theoretical premise the assessment is based. Since assessments are not pure and involve more than one area of human function, it is important to identify each of the areas.

8. Is normal behavior considered in the instrument? How is normal behavior scored? This important information tells the therapist how the client's results compare to those of the normal population.

9. Does the author tell you how to interpret the results? One must be able to translate results into treatment goals. This is the value of having results.

Research

A factor that cannot be overly emphasized is the need for research in the area of assessment development. This point is consistently important throughout this text. The last chapter is devoted to the research process in the development of assessments. However, the integrative approach can be used to generate research questions, from the selection process to treatment intervention. The integrative approach very clearly identifies differences in the treatment of clients, for example, in assessing social deficits. If a therapist believes that social deficits are environmental, the problems will be treated by one method. If a therapist believes that social deficits are caused by lack of skill, then the client will be treated by another method. The different methods can be applied to different clients to determine which method is most effective. This example may be over simplified, but it does illustrate the potential for the generation of research.

Summary

This chapter attempted to describe a structure that is dynamic in nature and reflective of the profession's domain of concern and legitimate tools. A visual structure that recognizes the aspects of human functions and allows the therapist to use a variety of assessments based on different theoretical premises was suggested. The literature review demonstrated that more than one theoretical premise can be used with a client. The central theme demonstrated that the eclectic approach was recognized as legitimate for occupational therapy.

The integrative structure is an eclectic approach influenced by clients' developmental tasks or milestones and cultural differences. It consists of four areas of human function— psychological, behavioral, learning, and biological—to which various frames of reference correspond. The term "area of human function" relate to Dunning's three modes. It is used to emphasize the unified wholeness of the individual. Humans are complex creatures whose behavior is influenced by the psychic, environment, skill acquisition, and physical health. They are interrelated and operate simultaneously. Health is a condition in which all four are operating harmoniously to achieve competence in occupational performances.

Listening is an important skill in the integrative approach to using assessments in mental health. Chapter II will go into detail about the role of listening in the occupational therapy process.

References

1. Conference Report (1968). Toward an integrated theory of occupational therapy. Am J Occup Ther 22, 451.
2. Owen CM (1968). An analysis of philosophy of occpational therapy. Am J Occup Ther 22, 502.
3. Dunning RE (1973). Philosophy and occupational therapy. Am J Occup Ther 27, 18.
4. Mosey AC (1970). Three Frames of Reference for Mental Health. Thorofare, New Jersey: Slack.
5. Mosey AC (1981). Occupational Therapy: Configuration of a Profession. New York: Raven Press.
6. Clark PN (1979). Human development through occupation; Theoretical frameworks in contemporary occupational therapy practice, Part 1. Am J Occup Ther 33, 505.
7. Kielhofner G and Burke JP (1980). A model of human occupation, Part 1, conceptual framework and content. Am J Occup Ther 34, 572.
8. Reed K (1984). Models of Practice in Occupational Therapy. Baltimore: Williams and Wilkins.
9. Azima M and Azima F (1959). Outline of a dynamic theory of occupational therapy. Am J Occup Ther 13, 215.
10. Fidler G and Fidler J (1967). Occupational Therapy: A Communicative Process. New York: MacMillan, 99-117.
11. Hemphill B (1982) B.H. Battery Training Manual. Thorofare, New Jersey: Slack.
12. Shoemyen C (1982). The Shoemyen battery, in Hemphill B (ed): The Evaluative Process in Psychiatric Occupational Therapy. Thorofare, New Jersey: Slack.
13. Evaskus M (1982) The Goodman battery, in Hemphill B (ed): The Evaluative Process in Psychiatric Occupational Therapy. Thorofare, New Jersey: Slack.
14. Lerner C (1982). The magazine picture collage, in Hemphill B (ed): The Evaluative Process in Psychiatric Occupational Therapy. Thorofare, New Jersey: Slack.
15. Mosey AC (1986). Psychosocial Components of Occupational Therapy. New York: Raven Press.

16. Keilhofner G (1985). A Model of Human Occupation: Theory and Application. Baltimore: Williams and Wilkins.
17. Barris R (1983). Psychosocial Occupational Therapy: In a Pleuristic Arena. Laurel, Maryland: RAMSCO.
18. Matsutsuyu J (1969). The interest checklist. Am J Occup Ther 23, 323-328.
19. Oakley F, Kielhofner G, Barris R, and Reicher R (1986).The role checklist: Development and empirical assessment of reliability. The Occupational Therapy Journal of Research 6(3):157.
20. Fidler G (1982). The lifestyle performance profile: An organizing frame, in Hemphill B (ed): The Evaluative Process in Psychiatric Occupational Therapy. Thorofare, New Jersey: Slack.
21. Spahn R. Paper presented at March 1965 meeting of the American Orthopsychiatric Society.
22. Black M (1976). Adolescent role assessment. Am J Occup Ther 30, 73-79.
23. Bloomer J and Williams S (1982). The BaFPE Administration Manual (2nd printing). Palo Alto, California: Consulting Psychologists Press.
24. Bloom BS et al (1956). Taxonomy of Educational Objectives Handbook 1: Cognitive Domain. New York: David McKay.
25. Harlow NJ (1971). Taxonomy of Psychomotor Domain. New York: David McKay.
26. Mosey AC (1973). Activities Therapy. New York: Raven Press.
27. McGourty L (1979). Kohlman Basic Living Skills Evaluation (2nd ed). Seattle: KELS Research.
28. Leonardelli C. Milwaukee Evaluation of Daily Living Skills. Unpublished manuscript.
29. Matheson L and Ogden L (1982). Work Capacity Evaluation. Rehabilitation Institute of Southern California.
30. Parachek J and King L (1982). Parachek Geriatric Rating Scale. Center for Neuro-developmental Studies.
31. King LJ (1974). A sensory-integrative approach to schizophrenia. Am J Occup Ther 28, 529.
32. Allen CK (1985). Occupational Therapy for Psychiatric Diseases: Measurement and Management of Cognitive Disabilities. Boston: Little, Brown.
33. Llorens LA (1977). A developmental theory revisited. Am J Occup Ther 31, 656.

34. Kielhofner G (1978). General systems theory; implications for theory and action in occupational therapy. Am J Occup Ther 32, 637.
35. Reed K and Sanderson SR (1980). Concepts of Occupational Therapy. Baltimore: Williams and Wilkins.

CHAPTER 2

LISTENING AS AN EVALUATIVE TOOL IN THE INTERVIEWING PROCESS

Barbara J. Hemphill, MS, OTR, FAOTA

Many of the occupational therapy assessments used in mental health include an interview as an integral part of the assessment.[1-9] If the interview is a part of an assessment and is standardized, the procedures are conducted according to instructions. The questions are closed and the interview is directive. However, most interviews in occupational therapy alternate from open-ended and client-centered, to closed with specific questioning. The purpose of the interview in most cases is for data gathering, problem identification, problem solving and goal setting for treatment.[10] The therapist asks questions and listens to the client's response. Listening is an important element in the interviewing process.[11] Moore[12] stated that listening provides the climate for communication in the occupational therapy interview.

The occupational therapist's primary focus in the interview is in four areas of human function.[13] The first is the intrapsychic nature of the individual, called the psychological area of human function. Such factors as reality contact, body concept, defense mechanisms, and impulse control are evaluated. The second is the behavioral area. This area concerns the individual's relationship with the environment and how random action is transformed into purposeful activity. The concept of reinforcement is examined by assessing the individual for maladaptive behavior that is reinforced by the human and non-human environment. The third area is learning. In this area the individual is assessed in skill acquisition. This includes activities of daily living, work skills, leisure skills, and cognitive skills. The last area of concern is biological. The therapist is concerned with the client's physical well-being.

In order to move from a systematic, structured, closed, directive, therapist-controlled interview to an open, non-directive, client-controlled interview designed to obtain information about client problems, the therapist must have a keen sense of listening. The therapist must not only be able to ask questions that reflect the areas of human function, but must be able to recognize, through a client's responses, the human function the client is expressing. A careful listener seeks transition from answers that lead to more questions.[14] In occupational therapy, the therapist must be able to respond to the client and be sensitive enough to identify transitions from one subject to another and from one area of human function to another. The act of listening to a client's responses is a vital ingredient of the communicative process in interviewing. The therapist must listen to what the client says, and how something is expressed. When the client is expressing an event, the therapist must listen to what is involved, where it occurred, or when it occurred. It is not only necessary to be effective senders, but to also be attentive receivers.[15]

The function of the interview as a part of the evaluative process was addressed in Chapter I. The purpose of this chapter is to examine listening as an integral part of the interview in occupational therapy assessment in mental health. A discussion of listening as related to the theory of communication will be proceeded by the techniques of listening in the interviewing process. The chapter will conclude with the implications for occupational therapy practice.

The Role of Listening in Communication

Listening as a Communicative Technique

Definition of Listening. Much of the data needed by helping persons to carry out their tasks is obtained in communication with clients. To make effective use of this data, helpers must learn to listen with great care to what the helpee is seeking to express. For clients, being listened to is much more than communication; it is a therapeutic experience in itself. For counselors, psychiatrists, social workers, and occupational therapists engaging in face-to-face communication with disturbed and troubled subjects, careful listening is an essential ingredient for successful practice.[15] Backland[16] stated that listening is recognized as an important skill, but researchers do not agree about its definition. However, several authors [12,17-19] identified components of listening.

The Components of Listening. The components of listening are thought to fall along a bipolar continuum.[17] At one end is a mental state characterized by alertness to external stimuli, acceptance of messages, and openness to input. The listener is attuned entirely to the client. The therapist gives full attention to the messages being received, imposing his or her own point of view only minimally. The key element is attentiveness, i.e., maintaining an external focus only on the client and on the message being transmitted.[18] Attending is probably the most powerful single communication skill in the interviewing process. Gazada, Childers and Walters[19] state that effective attending skills:

1. Are comfortable to use
2. Help caregivers listen and remember

3. Show interest in the talker

4. Do not work if used in a false and manipulative way because true feelings will be noticed

5. Look attractive from the talker's perspective

6. Increase the talker's feelings of trust and self-worth

7. Are a mark of respect for others

8. Have more impact on the talker than any other single communication skill (p. 103).

In the middle of the continuum is another mental state in which the listener is more actively selecting and organizing the material being received. The therapist is interested in information that is most essential in the client's message, what information is most personally relevant, and how the concepts are interrelated. The focus here is on understanding the message.[18] Understanding refers to the assignment of meaning to the messages received.[17]

At the far end of the continuum, the listener is weighing the message against personal beliefs, questioning the speaker's motives, challenging the ideas presented, suspecting the validity of the message, wondering what is being omitted, and in other ways evaluating what is said.[18] Listening involves hearing the way things are being said—and, what is not being said; that is, what is held under the surface.[12] This is called "listening with the third ear (page 193)."[15]

Listening with the third ear "involves attending to all that the client is expressing, not just verbally, but non-verbally as well, in his gestures, movements, inflections, even by what is specifically not said. Carl Rogers called the disciplined listening of helpers "non-evaluative listening (page 270)."[15]

When the therapist makes it easier for the client to discuss problems, to explore feelings, to gain understanding of the debilitating problem, and to build a therapeutic relationship, it is called facilitative communication.[19]

Gazda states:

"1. A facilitative response is one in which the helper verbally and non-verbally communicates what the professional has heard, what the helpee has said, and attempts to understand how the person feels.

2. Facilitative communication begins with thorough listening. Equally essential are the acts of reading the helpee's non-verbal messages while listening, synthesizing the communication received from the helpee.

3. A facilitative response is similar enough to the helpee's statement that the two could be interchanged. The helper's response communicates the content and affect of the helpee's statement with

accuracy and equal intensity. The helper does not add anything to what the helpee has said but also does not leave anything out (page 172)."

A Model for Listening

Miller[20] proposed a communication model that provides a framework for discussing listening as an important variable associated with interviewing. There are three major elements of the model. They are: a) a speaker, b) a listener, and c) feedback. The speaker sends (encodes) a message or asks a question as in an interview based on the interviewer's attitude. The message is decoded (translated) by the listener based on his attitudes. The listener gives positive and/or negative feedback to the interviewer in the form of answering the interviewer's questions. The interviewer then becomes the listener. The listener seeks understanding and allows the client to tell his story.[18,21]

Obstacles to Listening

Barker[17] identified three factors that could inhibit active listening. The first is inner conflict. People who have problems of a personal nature tend to devote considerable mental energy attempting to analyze their own problems. This mental preoccupation tends to interfere with listening. The second is general anxiety. Regardless of the origin of the anxiety, if it demanded a large proportion of the helpee's conscious thought time, it could decrease significantly a listener's effectiveness. The last factor is called closed-mindedness. Some individuals are open-minded selectively. That is, they are open-minded on those issues that are congruent with their own personal views.

Having reviewed some mental factors that inhibit listening, there are specific problems that could inhibit effective listening. The listening problems that relate to interviewing are: a) viewing what the client had to say as uninteresting, b) criticizing the speaker's delivery instead of the message, c) being ego-involved with the client's subject matter, d) listening only to facts, e) failing to adjust to distractions either by the client or distractions in the environment, f) faking attention, g) listening to what was easy to understand, h) allowing emotionally-laden words to interfere with listening, and i) permitting personal prejudices to impair comprehension and understanding.[17]

Suggestions to Improve Listening

Steil, Summerfield, and de Mare[22] discussed attitudes that improve listening. First is the willingness to not do all the talking.

The success of an interview may be directly proportional to the number of words spoken by the therapist.[12] The second attitude is that of warm acceptance of the person the therapist has agreed to listen to, and the ability to show this warmth in the manner and responsiveness of the therapist. "Facilitative responding provides a non-threatening atmosphere in which the helpee feels fully accepted and feels free to self-express in any manner the person chooses. In this atmosphere a relationship of mutual trust and caring can develop between helper and helpee (page 173)."[19]

Thirdly, is the attitude of making listening a part of the total communicative process.[22] Because of the nature of the therapeutic interview, the therapist has the obligation to give feedback to the client's responses to his inquiry in order to complete the communication cycle.[17]

Some additional approaches to improving listening are suggested by Steil, Summerfield, and de Mare[22] and supported by Barker.[17]

1. Maintain an attitude of objectivity. Keep an open mind

2. Focus on content of message, not delivery or physical mannerisms of the interviewee

3. Listen for main ideas, principles, concepts, not details

4. Try not to get "turned off" by specific phrases or "red flag" words

5. Be physically and mentally involved in the listening process [23]

6. Don't think about the next question while the interviewee is talking

7. Don't make value judgments until one has heard everything the interviewee has to say

8. Don't take notes word for word

9. Don't get mentally distracted.

The Role of Listening in Interviewing

Definition of Interviewing

Westhead[24] defines the interview as an exchange between two or more persons. That exchange is sometimes called "communication and it consists of both verbal and nonverbal messages." Littmann and Shugar[25] state that "interviewing is a procedure designed to help the interviewer toward a full understanding of the interviewee's situation."[81] The purposes are to obtain information, to give help, but mostly a combination of the two.[11] A successful medical interview has three main goals: a) to establish a positive physician-patient relationship, b) to elicit information about the patient's condition,[26] and c) to allow the interviewer to observe attitudes, feelings, and appearance[25]. It is a communicative process whereby the health professional uses interviewing to gather data upon which to base clinical decisions.[27]

Listening as a Technique in Interviewing

To be a good listener, one has to listen intently. This means concentrating on everything that is being said, how it is being said, and what is not being said.[25] The interviewer should be aware of shifts in conversation, recurrent references, inconsistencies and gaps, and concealed meaning.[11] Most researchers support the notion that listening is an important ingredient in interviewing clients.[11,15,16,18,19] The reasons that clients value the importance of listening are: a) the patients know more about their own bodily and mental health and can best describe each to the interviewer, b) the interviewer could make a premature diagnosis of the presenting problem if the client is not listened to, and c) the patient has the best knowledge about the history of the problem. When the client is listened to, it conveys the attitude that the relationship between the client and interviewer is a problem-solving venture.[21]

To enhance the listening process in the interview, Westhead[24] suggested some basic principles of communication. They are: a) mutual respect, b) acceptance of individual differences, c) shared openness, d) mutual perception of the problem, and e) conveyed shared concern, empathy, and steps toward a solution.

A productive method of obtaining specific information necessary for diagnosis and treatment, is asking questions that progress from the general to specific. The interviewer starts with a broad question, followed by a more detailed question. The question should be worded to elicit longer answers than "yes" or "no" responses. The client should do most of the talking.[26] The client should be solicited for opinions, thoughts, and feelings. This can be accomplished through indirect questioning.[28]

Specific techniques that communicate listening behavior to the client are proposed by Stano and Reinsch[29] and Westhead.[24]

1. Restatement—Repeat interviewee's words to make sure interviewee hears himself or for emphasis.

2. Rephrase—The interviewer alters the wording of a statement...so that the interviewer might better understand its meaning.

3. Probe—A more direct request for information.

4. Reflective—Restatement to convey understanding.

5. Clearinghouse—This is to let the interviewee volunteer relevant information which the interviewer has overlooked.

Other techniques suggested are agreement, elaboration, clarification, interpretation, and commenting on a non-verbal communication perceived as contradictory to verbal statements. In addition, commenting on two pieces of information that appear contradictory is important for an interviewer to use in an interview.[24] In clarification, the interviewer is submitting a synthesis of the interviewee's verbalized ideas and feeling for approval. In interpretation, the interviewer is responding to the interviewee's frame of reference and life space.[28]

Discussion and Summary

Implications for Occupational Therapy

Interviewing is an integral part of the evaluative process in assessing client functioning for occupational therapy in mental health. The purpose of the interview as an evaluative tool is to identify and solve clients' problems, gather data for further evaluation and set goals for treatment. For the most part, when an assessment is accompanied with an interview, the questions are asked in a standardized way. This leaves little opportunity for clients to offer their own interpretation of the problem. The interview is fact finding, therapist controlled, and devoid of client interaction. However, because of the nature of the information needed for client treatment, it is necessary that the interview in occupational therapy alternate between asking specific questions and asking open-ended questions. This allows the clients to express themselves, to express feelings, to explain the problem in their own words, and to add information that would not be included in a standardized interview. In order to accomplish this, a system for integrating occupational therapy knowledge and a structure from which to approach the interview is suggested by Hemphill.[13]

The integrative approach recognizes the aspects of human function described by Hemphill.[13] In order to conduct an interview that examines all the aspects of human function and how they are related to each other, it is necessary to have a keen sense of listening skills. The questions must reflect the aspects of human function in order to get information about each of the modes. However, the therapist must listen to the client's response to determine which human function the client is expressing. Therefore, the therapist must listen to transitions made by the client and be able to respond to the client. In this sense, the client is leading the therapist in the interview. But the therapist must respond appropriately in order to obtain information about the client's problems.

Therefore, listening is an important element in the occupational therapy interview. It provides a climate for communication. For clients, being listened to is much more than mere communication; it is a therapeutic experience. Listening is recognized as an important skill in interviewing, but researchers do not agree about its definition. There is some agreement about the components of listening. They are: a) attending, b) understanding the message, and c) evaluating what is said.

When the therapist makes it easier for clients to discuss their problems, to explore feelings, to build a therapeutic relationship, client needs can be analyzed and treatment planned. Because interviewing is more than listening and listening is communication that enhances a therapeutic climate for client treatment, this author suggests that the training of students for occupational therapy include the development of listening skills. Also, this author suggests that workshops be offered to practicing therapists as continuing education. The need for this is apparent in a study by Moore.[12] The author stated that the data suggest that the client is forced into a path of giving information, responding to specific questions, and revealing little about himself. Training in how to listen would enhance the interview as an evaluative tool in occupational therapy.

Miller suggested that the communication model be used to provide a framework for learning to listen. The emphasis should be on asking questions that alternate between specific and general. The feedback received in the form of client responses also should be emphasized. The student should be taught how to use techniques such as restating, rephrasing, probing, reflecting, clearinghouse, elaborating, clarifying, and interpreting.

Summary

The purpose of this chapter was to examine listening as an integral part of the interview in occupational therapy mental health. It is agreed that to make effective use of the data obtained in the interview, helpers must learn to listen because an interview is more than just sharing information; it is a therapeutic experience. Even though there is no agreement on the definition of listening, most researchers agree on the components of listening. The components of listening are thought to fall along a bipolar continuum. Attending is probably the most powerful single communication skill in the interviewing process. In the middle of the continuum, the listener focuses on understanding the message. At the far end of the continuum, the listener is involved in hearing the way things are being said and what is not being said. A model for listening is discussed which emphasizes a) the speaker, b) the listener, and c) the feedback.

Three factors that are obstacles to listening are inner conflict, general anxiety, and closed-mindedness. Some specific problems are: a) viewing clients as uninteresting, b) being ego-involved, c) faking attention d) listening only to facts, and e) permitting personal prejudices to interfere in understanding. Attitudes to improve listening include letting the client do all the talking, warm acceptance of the client, and making listening a part of the total communicative process in the interview.

Interviewing is defined as communication between two persons which consists of both verbal and non-verbal messages. The purpose is toward a combination of obtaining information and giving help. It is a communicative process whereby the helping professional uses interviewing to gather data upon which to base clinical decisions. Interviewing requires good listening techniques.

To be a good listener one must listen intently. The therapist must listen to everything that is being said, how it is said, and what is not said. One should be aware of shifts in conversation, recurrent references, inconsistencies, gaps and concealed meaning. In order to listen, there are some basic principles of communication. They are: a) mutual respect, b) acceptance of individual differences, c) shared openness, d) mutual perception of the problem, and e) shared concern. Questions must progress from the general to specific, followed by a more broad question. Techniques that communicate listening behavior to the client are: a) restatement, b) rephrase, c) probe, d) reflective, and e) clearinghouse.

References

1. Androes L, Dryfus E, and Bloesch M (1965). Diagnostic test battery for occupational therapy. Am J Occup Ther 19, 53.
2. Black M (1976). Adolescent role assessment. Am J Occup Ther 30, 73.
3. Bloomer J and Williams S (1982). The Bay area functional performance evaluation, in Hemphill B (ed): The Evaluative Process in Psychiatric Occupational Therapy. Thorofare, New Jersey: Slack.
4. Florey L and Michelman S (1982). Occupational role history: A screening tool for psychiatric occupational therapy. Am J Occup Ther 36, 301.

5. Hemphill B (1980). Mental health evaluations used in occupational therapy. Am J Occup Ther 34, 721.

6. McGourty L (1979). Kohlman Evaluation of Living Skills. Unpublished manuscript.

7. Mosey AC (1973). Activities Therapy. New York: Raven Press.

8. Peters M and Clark N (1982). The Scorable Self Care Evaluation. Thorofare, New Jersey: Slack.

9. Pezzuti L (1979). An exploration of adolescent feminine and occupational behavior development. Am J Occup Ther 33, 84.

10. Shaw C (1982). The interview process, in Hemphill B (ed): The Evaluative Process in Psychiatric Occupational Therapy. Thorofare, New Jersey: Slack.

11. Garrett A (1972). Interviewing: Its Principles and Methods (2nd ed). New York: Family Service Association of America.

12. Moore JW (1977). The initial interview and interaction analysis. Am J Occup Ther 31, 29-33.

13. Hemphill B (ed) (1982). The Evaluative Process in Psychiatric Occupational Therapy. Thorofare, New Jersey: Slack.

14. Wolff F, Marsnik N, Tacey W, and Michols R (1983). Perceptive Listening. New York: Holt, Rinehart and Winston.

15. Combs A, Avila D, and Purkey W (1972). Helping Relationships: Basic Concepts for the Helping Professions. Boston: Allyn and Bacon, 269.

16. Backland P (1983). Methods of assessing speaking and listening skills, in Rubin RB (ed): Improving Speaking and Listening Skills. San Francisco: Jossey-Bass, 70.

17. Barker LL (1971). Listening Behavior. Englewood Cliffs, New Jersey: Prentice-Hall.

18. Friedman P (1978). Listening Processes: Attention, Understanding, Evaluation. Washington D.C.: National Education Association.

19. Gazda G, Childers W, and Walters R (1982). Interpersonal Communication: A Handbook for Health Professionals. Rockville, Maryland: Aspen.

20. Miller G (1972). An Introduction to Speech Communication. New York: Bobbs Merrill.

21. DiMatteo M and Friedman M (1982). Social Psychology and Medicine. Cambridge, Massachusetts: Oelgeschlager, Gunn, and Hain Publishers, Inc.

22. Steil L, Summerfield J, and de Mare G (1983). Listening: It Can Change Your Life. New York: John Wiley and Sons.

23. Wolvin AD (1983). Improving listening skills, in Rubin RB (ed): Improving Speaking and Listening Skills. San Francisco: Jossey-Bass, 17.
24. Westhead E (1978). Interviewing: An abbreviated introduction. Academic Therapy 13(3):329.
25. Littmann S and Gerald Shugar G (1980). The examination: History, in Greben S, Pos R, Rakoff V, Bonkalo A, Lowy F, and Voineskos G (eds): A Method of Psychiatry. Philadelphia: Lea and Febiger.
26. Bernstein L and Bernstein R (1985). Interviewing: A Guide for Health Professionals (4th ed). New York: Appleton-Century-Crofts.
27. Enelow A and Swisher S (1972). Interviewing and Patient Care. New York: Oxford University Press.
28. Benjamin A (1981). The Helping Interview (3rd ed). Boston: Houghton Mifflin.
29. Stano M and Reinsch N (1982). Communication in Interviews. Englewood Cliffs, New Jersey: Prentice-Hall.

CHAPTER 3

THE INTERVIEWING PROCESS IN OCCUPATIONAL THERAPY

Carol Shaw, MA, OTR

The ability to interview is a necessary and fundamental skill which must be acquired by the occupational therapist. It is the primary mode of communication through which the therapist is able to understand and ultimately help another human being. Interviewing is a skill that can be improved through constant practice, the acquisition of knowledge regarding the theory of human psychodynamics and the principles and concepts of interviewing, and the conscious and constant examination of one's own interviewing.

This chapter will attempt to provide the reader with some basic information about the interviewing process. The interview will be defined and its purposes will be discussed as it relates to the evaluation process in occupational therapy. Information will be presented on how to conduct an interview as well as some potential problems in interviewing. Specific occupational therapy evaluations administered by the interviewer will be reviewed. Techniques and approaches for interviewing difficult patients will also be addressed briefly.

Definition of an Interview

As defined by Sullivan,[1] an interview is a situation in which two or more people verbally communicate with each other about a particular subject matter for a specific purpose. The subject matter and specific purpose(s) are determined by the individuals involved and the nature of the setting or facility in which the interview is taking place. As the "expert" in the field of interpersonal relationships and behavior, it is the therapist's responsibility to identify the needs of the interviewee and how the client will benefit from their interchange. It is imperative to focus on two basic concepts as one begins to conduct an interview. These concepts are: 1) to discover what the needs of the client are, and 2) how best to help or benefit the client. With these two ideas in mind, many of the problems and anxiety-producing situations of the occupational therapist can be reduced.

Purposes of the Interview

Occupational therapists are required to interview clients. Throughout the entire occupational therapy process, in order to evaluate and treat, one must gather information, identify problems, problem solve, goal set for treatment and discharge of the client. It is the evaluation process and subsequent treatment plan that distinguishes a professional or occupational therapist from an arts-and-crafts person or an activity worker.

The interview is a primary technique in both these processes of evaluation and treatment. As a brief review, the following ideas are presented.

Data Gathering—Data gathering is the first component in the evaluation process. The interview with the client serves as the primary source of data. Other sources include, but are not limited to, the client's family and significant others, the client's chart, and other helping professions working with the client. Through collecting data, the reliability and validity of previously gathered information can be checked. One must only gather information needed to help the client, not to satisfy one's own curiosity. Know the reason a question is being asked. It is important to remember that the purpose of the interview needs to be shared and mutually understood by both parties involved. This mutual understanding will generally facilitate the accomplishment of the goals of the interviewer. Finally, the setting or facility in which the interview takes place influences the nature and amount of information sought.

Problem Identification—Problem identification is another important purpose of the interview process. Here one identifies the problems, strengths, limitations, and resources of the client. An occupational therapist must understand the problems the client is experiencing and their possible causes before attempting intervention. Mutual identification of the difficulties must also take place in order for the therapist and client to become actively involved in a therapeutic alliance. If mutual identification of the problems does not occur, the client and therapist may be working at odds with each other. When, where, and how these problems in living occur must also be identified.

Problem Solving—In the problem-solving process, it is the accurate and precise identification of a problem which is the crucial first step. It is only after accomplishing this first step that the occupational therapist and client can begin to determine what additional information is needed and where, how, or from whom this information is to be obtained.

Goal Setting—Another purpose of interviewing is one of goal setting for treatment. Here the interviewer focuses on the development of goals and objectives for the treatment plan and the therapeutic relationship. Again, this must be a mutual process in which both parties collaborate and agree upon the goals and objectives of treatment. Generally, goal setting is done systematically or informally.

Final Interview—The final interview in the occupational therapy process has several purposes. An overview of what has occurred in the course of treatment may be the focus of this interview. The overview may serve to reinforce learning that has already taken place or help delineate potential problems or concerns that might be experienced by the client in the near future.

Content of an Interview

The factual information given by the interviewee is one aspect making up the content of the interview. It is that content that is readily accessible to the client or interviewee. It includes thoughts, feelings, and experiences about the past, present, and future life experiences, situations, and plans of the client. This is material that can be validated quite easily by the occupational therapist. This information was labeled introspective data by MacKinnon and Micheals.[2] This introspective data is essentially how the client views particular situations, problems, strengths, or limitations. It also serves in part to give the interviewer some ideas regarding the client's level of motivation, insight, energies, and resources available to address problems.

The interview also provides other information called inspective data. Inspective data is the non-verbal behavior of the interviewer and the interviewee.[2] Usually the client does not know or understand the important and significant messages or data which are being communicated on a non-verbal level. It is the occupational therapist's responsibility to know, analyze, and use this non-verbal data to help understand what ails the client. Therefore, content involves both the verbal and non-verbal behaviors of the interviewer and interviewee.

The interviewer may be able to infer through observing the client's motor behavior more definitive and specific ideas or thoughts than may have been expressed verbally. For example, a client who plays with a bracelet or ring is communicating more than a generalized feeling of anxiety or discomfort. It is this sensitivity, awareness, and understanding of non-verbal communication that enables the interviewer to observe, listen to, and thereby ascertain the emotional state of the client. In order to understand these disguised messages, the therapist must strive to develop the "third ear." Initially described by Theodore Reik,[3] the third ear refers to the therapist's ability to sense on a conscious level what the client is unconsciously communicating.

The third ear works in essentially two ways. First, it "hears" what people do not say, that is, what they feel and think, and secondly, the third ear listens to what is being heard or felt by the therapist. Through this processing, the information provided by the client is integrated with the previous knowledge and emotions of the therapist's unconscious. It is then brought back to the therapist's consciousness after the significance of what the client has said has been made meaningful. This skill is one that is difficult to teach. It requires that the therapist be open and sensitive to the more subtle nuances and more fleeting and elusive communications of the client.[3] The therapist needs to become sensitive to what is not present, as well as what is present and expected. The therapist is, in essence, being sensitive to the hidden or concealed communication that the client is conveying.

Process of the Interview

The process of an interview is an important source of information. Process is defined here as any change in the relationship of the interviewer and interviewee. The process usually can be noted when there is a change in the attitude of the interviewee or in the attitude of the interviewer, which is usually reflected or mirrored back in the client's attitude. This latter change is often difficult for the interviewer to notice and requires a greater effort on his part.

Why is it important to notice, examine, and then hopefully understand the process of an interview? The answer lies in the belief that the manner in which an individual interacts with another person is characteristic of and reflects his skill in interpersonal relationships.

The following questions are offered to help the reader begin the process of analyzing an interview:

Did I speak too rapidly, professionally, or glibly? When and for what possible reasons did I have to redirect or refocus the course of the interview?

Why did the client interrupt me at that particular moment? How did the client act towards me or vice versa—charming, hostile, or evasive?

What made me ask that certain question or make that comment at that particular time?

What about the client made me phrase my questions in a particular manner?

The above questions are only a sample of the type of questioning and analysis that will enable the interviewer to examine the process of an interview. These questions and answers require the therapist to have a great deal of self-awareness and the ability to see himself objectively. As a beginning occupational therapist, there are also several tools or clues which will enable an easier analysis of an interview. These tools are:

1. Shifts in conversation, either by the therapist or the patient. While the connection or relationship between the subjects is immediately unclear, some connection does generally exist and needs only to be discovered.

2. Repeated themes are generally of great importance to the patient, but also potentially do not permit other areas of the patient's life to be explored. It is important, especially in the evaluation process, to obtain facts and understand the many aspects of the patient's life and not just one or two areas of concern.

3. Gaps are important clues to better understanding of the patient. Gaps in historical information time or relationships may indicate lack of development, experience, or knowledge in the omitted area of living. Again, it is important information to obtain during the evaluation process.

4. Inconsistencies also may be utilized as a tool to examine the changes or attitudes that occur during the interview. Inconsistencies in information may point to anxiety, conflict, or confusion.

5. Hidden meanings provide the therapist with valuable clues about the client's problems. It is crucial that one attempts to listen with the third ear.

Problems in Communication

Most problems in communication stem from anxiety. Anxiety generally occurs when a person's self-esteem or self-regard is being threatened. While a moderate amount of anxiety is often useful, anxiety may become unproductive when it overwhelms the individual. Anxiety affects both the interviewer and interviewee. It is, however, the therapist's responsibility to recognize behaviors resulting from anxiety. A few examples of such behaviors include, but are certainly not limited to, irrational anger, misunderstandings of meanings, misinterpretations, lateness, pressured or rapid speech, confusion, authority acting, judgmental attitudes, talking up, down, or around an issue, using professional jargon, and using words or phrases the other person is not familiar with. The list is endless and includes behaviors of both the interviewer and interviewee. Both parties are susceptible to acting out felt anxiety. It is, however, the occupational therapist's responsibiliy to avoid arousing unnecessary anxiety in the client. While a moderate amount of anxiety can be productive, generation of anxiety only should be used when it is clearly in the best interest of the client.

In most instances, the occupational therapist needs to act in such a way as to restrain the development of anxiety within the interviewee. It is often helpful to reassure the client that some anxiety is natural and generally diminishes as the interview proceeds. As an inexperienced therapist, one's own anxiety may lead to obstacles in communication. Some possible pitfalls might be talking or using language unfamiliar to the interviewee, using professional jargon, coming on like an authority figure, or allowing interruptions to occur during the interview. By allowing interruptions to occur or by not ending them quickly, the interviewer is giving a clear, implicit message, i.e., "This interview situation is making me uncomfortable, because I'm anxious, or bored, etc." Repeated interruption of the client probably will result in the client's giving up trying to talk. It is clear from the interviewer's behavior that he is not really listening to the client.

The judging of another person's behavior or attitude is oftentimes a result of anxiety. As an interviewer, one might describe the client as uncooperative, a troublemaker, and/or eccentric. These judgments tend to limit one's own self-reflection and evaluation of self-behavior in the interview. It also tends to "pigeon-hole" the client into a certain category or classification. What will be missing is a true understanding of the client. Acquiring this real understanding of the client is important and necessary. The more information compiled and the further the understanding, the greater is one's potential ability to help the client.

Types of Interviews in the Evaluative Process

In the evaluative process, the occupational therapist uses many different evaluation procedures. Each procedure uses some type of interviewing process or technique. There are several different ways of classifying or describing these types of interviews. One classification system states that interviewers may be understood along a continuum from structured to unstructured. Most, if not all the evaluations used by occupational therapists may be placed somewhere along this continuum: structured, semi-structured, and unstructured.

A structured interview is designated as standardized and addresses a specific area of concern or interest. In standardized interviews, similar information is gathered from different people and is compared and classified. Similarities and differences in the answers given are noted and may reflect similarities and differences in the interviewees and not in the questions. A structured interview is one in which there are predetermined questions and fixed responses with which the interviewee may respond. There is little room to explore further information or clarification.

In psychiatric occupational therapy, only one evaluation procedure to date has been standardized and uses a structured interview. This is the evaluation procedure, the Bay Area Functional Performance Evaluation (BaFPE) developed by Bloomer and Williams.[4] This evaluation has a predetermined sequence of questions and experiences which may not be altered. Interpretation of scoring against normative scales is utilized.

In the semi-structured interview, predetermined specific questions are also used to gather information about an area of concern. However, in the semi-structured interview, the interviewer is permitted to ask other questions in order to clarify or probe for more information. There is generally a schedule of questions or a general outline of the information being sought which assists the interviewer in this data collection.

In the area of psychiatric occupational therapy, a majority of the evaluation procedures currently used fall into the semi-structured category. For instance, the Occupational History,[5] Interest Checklist,[6] and the Activities Configuration[7] use the semi-structured interview as the primary mode of obtaining information or clarification of information.

In the unstructured or unstandardized interview, there are no predetermined questions. The interviewer explores whatever phenomena seems most crucial, useful, or pertinent to the interests of the interviewee. This type of interview requires great skill in the interview process and sensitivity to the client, for it allows the occupational therapist to explore material or matters that are interesing, but may be irrelevant to the purpose of the interview.

Most of the projective evaluative procedures used in occupational therapy fall into the unstructured category. The tasks, i.e., purpose of the interview, are predetermined; the questions and areas of exploration are left up to the therapist and/or client to define. In these types of evaluations, it is crucial that the interviewer use skills in interviewing to facilitate exploration of the issues and concerns that arise.

Naturally, an interview may contain all these types of questions or formats. For instance, a "structured section" of an interview asks for the name, address, date of birth, etc. Another segment of the same interview might center around an activity or work schedule or an interest checklist. This would be an example of a semi-structured interview. An unstructured segment of the interview would be the exploration of the interviewee's work relationship or past interests or activities.

Basic Components of a Helping Interview

In conducting a successful helping interview, the occupational therapist must possess skills in the basic components of an interview. These components are essential in both evaluation and treatment interviews. The components— listening, observing, questioning, and responding to the client—will be addressed and described here. The reader is urged to delve in greater depth and detail in the volumes of books written on these components.

Listening

Listening is the single most important and fundamental component in the interviewing process. As stated by Balinsky and Burger,[8] the "biggest block to personal communication is man's inability to listen intelligently, understandingly and skillfully to another person." Listening is an act of giving which demands a temporary "unconcern" for oneself (page 38).[8]

Listening requires both mental and emotional functions. A good listener tries to think where the interview is headed and is able to act as a mirror and sounding board that throws back a reflection to the interviewee, thus providing the speaker with an opportunity to see and hear in a way otherwise not possible. It is a difficult skill to learn and requires constant effort to perfect.

Listening is an active, complex, and tiring process. One cannot sit back and let the interviewee talk. If this is done, a real opportunity to know the other person is lost. Knowing the other person means understanding how he thinks and feels about himself and how he thinks and feels about others in the world; how he sees others relating to him; what his goals, hopes, and plans are for the future; how he copes with problems; what defense mechanisms he uses; and what his belief system is. Because listening is such an active process, and because we are all humans, there will be lapses in attention. Oftentimes, these lapses are "caused by" the interviewee repeating or by the interviewer having an internal dialogue with himself.

Good listening is a selective process. A good listener is someone who is actively attentive to the general, recurrent or major themes of the interviewee, rather than to details. A good listener also searches for the message between the lines. (See discussion on the "third ear.") This selective effort requires that the occupational therapist be clear about the purpose for which he is listening. This purpose or goal allows him to screen out what is not necessary information. For example, in trying to determine the reasons for the client's repeated arguments with the teacher, the occupational therapist may need to pay close attention to the client's description of his relationship with fellow students and classmates, as well as his relationship with that teacher.

Observing

Observation is another important and fundamental component in conducting an interview. Observation is defined as the active noticing or seeing that occurs continuously throughout the interview. Observation is influenced by one's expectations or one's psychological set. In an article that appeared in the *American Journal of Occupational Therapy*, students' observations of the same subject were reported to be significantly altered due to the information given to them prior to their observations.[9] Thus, as with listening, it is essential to be somewhat ignorant in an effort to reduce or eliminate to as great a degree as possible any biases or preconceptions. This is an important point and should be given serious consideration as one learns to interview and learns from experiences.

A great deal has been written about body language and non-verbal communication. The use of activities and other modes of non-verbal communication in the occupational therapy evaluation and treatment process makes it absolutely essential that the occupational therapist be knowledgeable in this form of communication. As non-verbal communication is more primitive, it is more reliable than verbal clues or messages. As with verbal messages, non-verbal communications must be validated. One cannot interpret a non-verbal message, such as lip biting, and label it a sign of anxiousness, or decide that tongue movement is a neurological symptom without first validating the message. One must view non-verbal communication in the context of the situation, being extremely careful not to draw firm conclusions without validating the meaning of the non-verbal communication with the client.

Questioning

Asking questions is another critical component in conducting an interview. What questions to ask and how and when to ask these questions are crucial issues with the beginning occupational therapist. If one asks too many questions, a pattern of interaction is established with the client which will be difficult to change. However, one is also faced with the responsibility and need to elicit certain information from the interviewee.

The problem of what questions to ask is often solved if one is clear about the purpose of the interview. The purpose of the interview will influence the information sought and will therefore shape the nature of the questions asked.

Another determinant in the evaluative interview is the type and specific evaluation tool or procedure used. Questions should be asked that are relevant and pertinent to the problems of the client, rather than those that will satisfy the curiosity of the therapist.

The actual types of questions asked (i.e., open-ended or closed-ended) will depend on the nature of the information sought. Open-ended questions are most useful in eliciting more emotionally laden responses, as they allow the client to respond more freely. Closed-ended questions are used more often when focusing on more factual information. For instance, an example of an open-ended question might be, "How did you feel when you lost your job?" An example of a closed-ended question might be, "When did you lose your job?"

Questions should be asked when something has been missed that the client has said or to assess whether or not the client has understood something in the interview. One may also want to explore a particular area or issue more fully and clarify what the event actually means. The client may need help in clarifying or exploring a thought or feeling and a question would help to refocus his thoughts. There are also occasions when the topic or feeling that the interviewee is discussing is a particularly difficult one for him to verbalize. A question asked with a supportive, understanding attitude may encourage the client to discuss it. For example, "It seems like a difficult topic. Is there something else about this subject that makes it a difficult one for you?"

Questions must be asked in a facilitating way. Too often the beginning occupational therapist will ask too many questions at once. This barrage of questions is linked more closely to the therapist's own anxiety level than to seeking information. Ill-timed questions can effectively confuse the client by interrupting concentration. Questions that force or impel the person to choose between two items or answers should be avoided. For instance, asking someone, "did you go to college or work at a job?" leaves them little opportunity to tell what actually happened during that particular time period. Finally, avoid asking, "why" too often. It's an extremely difficult question for most of us to answer, and many people do not know why they behave or feel a certain way. The question also has a punitive connotation which will not facilitate a free flow of communication.

The purpose of asking a question is to obtain an answer. Therefore, once a question is asked, stop, wait, and listen to the answer. All too often while interviewing, one thinks ahead in one's mind to the next question before the client has finished answering. If the client begins to answer questions curtly and too quickly, it behooves the therapist to identify if active listening is taking place.

Response of the Interviewer

The verbal and non-verbal responses that are given during an interview will determine to a great extent the client's comfort and willingness to share thoughts and feelings. The responses will convey the attitude, level of interest, concern, and understanding. Hopefully, verbal responses will help the interviewee understand both him-or herself and others more closely and clarify feelings and thoughts about life situation.

The kinds of possible verbal responses are practically limitless. The most frequently used and described in the literature on interviewing are the following:

1. A minimal verbal response is the "uh-huh," "mm-mm," or "yes" utterances or head nods of the occupational therapist that give the client the sense of being listened to and understood.

2. In paraphrasing, the main purpose is to reflect back to the client what he has said, to demonstrate to the client that the interviewer understands what is being said or to stress one particular component or phrase of the client's statement.

3. Reflection deals primarily with the unstated or implied feelings or concerns of the interviewee. The occupational therapist must be able to accurately assess the feeling, tone, and attitude of the client and to verbalize these feelings and attitudes in a clear and acceptable manner to the client.

4. To probe, one generally uses an open-ended statement which attempts to gain more information about a particular subject, issue, or feelings. Clarification of the information can occur for both parties in an interview. Responses of the occupational therapist may be geared to help clarify something for the client or for the therapist. In the first instance, the occupational therapist might attempt

to refocus or express something about which the interviewee is confused or is having difficulty expressing. In the latter instance, the occupational therapist needs to have something clarified for his own understanding of what is being discussed.

5. Confrontation involves the occupational therapist giving honest feedback to the client about how the therapist really sees what is happening to the client.

Interviewing Difficult Patients

As previously stated, successful interviewing requires in-depth knowledge regarding the theories of human psychodynamics. These theories are established around certain basic assumptions. One such assumption is that all behavior is purposeful or goal directed and is a product or result of some hypothetical force, i.e., drives, urges, impulses, or motives. These forces manifest themselves in a subjective manner through one's thoughts and feelings and objectively through patterns of behavior or action. Knowledge based on some theoretical framework of these motivating forces enables the interviewer to better understand both the dynamics of the interview situation and the psychodynamics of the client.

While it might be interesting to delve more deeply into other aspects of human psychodynamic theories, it is not feasible within the scope of this chapter to do so. Therefore, the reader is urged to become well-versed in these theories and areas of knowledge in order to develop skills.

The remainder of this section will focus on three major clinical syndromes frequently present in difficult clients being interviewed. Again, the author's assumption is that the reader has a well-grounded knowledge of the syndrome's psychodynamic patterns, clinical features, and precautions. Three types of patients will be addressed: the depressed patient, the schizophrenic patient, and the paranoid or hostile patient. Some suggestions will be given regarding the management and structure of interviews with these patients.

The Depressed Patient

The depressed patient's major clinical symptoms involve a lowering of mood and a loss of interest in life. Generally, appetite for food diminishes and the patient finds little in life to enjoy. Feelings of anxiety are often present, which may ultimately be replaced by apathy and withdrawal. The patient's thoughts primarily concern his own problems. He mulls over and over thoughts about the past and is generally guilt ridden and hopeless.

With the depressed patient, the interviewer needs to become an active participant in the interview process. The interviewer must provide structure for the interview and, to some extent, gratify the dependent needs of the depressed patient. In general, this type of patient has a low energy level and in actuality may not be able to engage in the interview process actively. The entire interview will be slow and the interviewer needs to allow time for responses. One needs to maintain a supportive, reassuring, and concerned manner. It is useful to be aware that one's own anxiety may interfere with the interview process. If one finds oneself being too upbeat, cheerful, or energetic and rapid, one's anxiety is showing. Slow down. This increase of energy or elevated mood on the part of the interviewer may give the client a message of the interviewer's inability to tolerate the client's depression. If a depressed patient wants to express unhappiness, it is necessary to allow him to do so.

A depressed patient does not become emotionally involved with the interviewer as do other clients. This emotional silence is often difficult to overcome and may need to be addressed in a supportive, concerned manner. One might comment, "talking seems to be a difficult thing for you to do." If the interviewer remains silent and offers no encouragement or support, the depressed patient may view this behavior as disinterest, dissatisfaction or frustration, reinforcing a sense of failure and hopelessness.

Most moderately depressed patients cry, while most severely or chronically depressed patients rarely do. If a client does cry during an interview, it is useful to be supportive and sympathetic, perhaps by offering a tissue or, depending on the relationship between the interviewer and client, gently touching the patient on the shoulder or knee and waiting for the crying to subside. Then begin the interview again—neither too quickly, nor too late. One good indication of the "right" time is once the client has blown his nose, wiped his eyes, or looked at the interviewer.

One last area of concern in interviewing the depressed patient has to do with the potential and real threat of suicide. While it is often difficult for new therapists to deal with the issues of suicide, it is of utmost importance to address and understand whatever, if any, suicidal thoughts are present in the depressed patient. Knowing their thoughts often helps in determining the severity and danger of their depression. Sometimes simple, direct questions may help to decrease the client's anxiety.[2] If the client reports such feelings and thoughts to the therapist, it is crucial to share this information with the treating professionals.

The Schizophrenic Patient

Interviewing the schizophrenic patient is a difficult, challenging experience. The schizophrenic suffers from disturbances in the four major areas of psychological functioning. To review, there are disturbances in affect, thoughts, behavior, and interpersonal relationships. As a result of these disturbances, there is a great deal of variety and difference in the symptoms manifested by different patients. Also, one patient may, through the course of a lifetime, show a great variety of symptoms. These symptoms reflect the emotional life of the schizophrenic patient and therefore need to be understood in terms of significance to the patient. While the patient's feelings may seem inappropriate either to the situation or to expressed thoughts, these emotional responses are internally consistent.[2] That is, they are appropriate to the patient's inner-life experiences. The disturbances in the affective areas oftentimes lead to estrangement from others. The schizophrenic patient is unable to engage comfortably in an emotional life with others and is also unable to find pleasure in the solitude that results.

The disturbances in thought experienced by the schizophrenic patient are not random. The patient's ideas may come out in a confusing and often bewildering manner, but may be understandable in the context of inner experiences. One possible way of understanding the patient's disturbed thoughts is to view them as serving a purpose. That is, the thought disorganization helps to, on an unconscious level, defend against some emerging anxiety or obscure an uncomfortable topic. When interviewing the schizophrenic patient, one also needs to be aware of the patient's decreased attention span and the difficulty in shifting from one topic to another. The schizophrenic patient may also demonstrate an inability to comprehend the various meanings of a particular word. The patient may become quite literal and concrete in his understanding and subsequent responses. For example, the patient may answer literally, "the bus," to the interviewer's question regarding what got him to the hospital.

One final area of concern and interest regarding the patient's thought processes is fantasy. The schizophrenic patient spends a great deal of time preoccupied with fantasies and may, in fact, lose the ability to differentiate fantasy from reality. Fantasy is for the schizophrenic, as it is for all of us, an attempt to retreat from reality and solve some problems. However, as stated previously, the schizophrenic patient may not be sure where fantasy stops and reality begins. For this reason, exploration of the schizophrenic patient's fantasy life is contraindicated in the evaluation phase of treatment, as it may further decrease the patient's contact with reality.

The behavior of the schizophrenic is often characterized by apathy. Indeed, the schizophrenic patient generally lacks initiative and motivation and will appear bored and listless.

Again, it is necessary to examine the dynamics of this behavior. One may understand this lack of initiative and motivation as the patient's attempt to avoid the discomfort or anxiety resulting from another potential 'failure' situation. The schizophrenic patient may also manifest behavior which is often disorganized, inappropriate and ambivalent in its goal direction. For example, a patient requests placement in a prevocational group which requires punctuality for admittance. The patient then comes late to her other groups for several days prior to placement, thus revealing ambivalent feelings regarding increased commitment and responsibility.

The final area of disturbance is in interpersonal relationships. The schizophrenic patient has difficulty in relating to and trusting others. While much has been written about this area, it is the mistrust, fear of closeness, ambivalance and clinging dependence of the schizophrenic patient which characterize and impact on all his human interactions.

These qualities also will be apparent in the interview situation. This must be recognized and understood by the therapist. It is very difficult to establish a meaningful emotional rapport with the schizophrenic patient. The client's mistrust and fear of closeness and engulfment will lead him to protect himself through isolation and withdrawal. It is therefore useful and facilitating of the therapist to structure and clearly define the scope and content of the interview while allowing the patient to feel as though his needs are being met.

One of the most common problems encountered in interviewing is the schizophrenic patient's use of disorganization as a defense.[2] When asked a question, the schizophrenic patient will start to answer and then either shift or change to another topic or else remain on the same topic, but the words and sentences will be confusing. It is important at these times that the interviewer, instead of withdrawing or trying to conceal over boredom, offer the patient support and reveal difficulty in understanding the patient. By simply saying, "I'm having difficulty following what you are saying," the interviewer is offering a supportive response and one which is preferable to a more accusatory statement, such as, "You're not being clear."

With the schizophrenic patient it is often useful to offer some structure to the interview situation. For instance, one might explain the purpose of a particular evaluation and how its results might relate to the patient's own problems. Many times schizophrenics may, in fact, not be able to articulate the areas of function in which they are having difficulties. Here again it would be helpful to offer some supportive and directive suggestions. For example, if the patient reports about difficulty finding a job, the interviewer may try to pinpoint where in the process of job hunting he is having difficulty and the specific nature of the difficulty.

Interviewing the schizophrenic requires an enormous amount of patience, and a great deal of empathy for someone who is suffering profoundly. While it is often a frustrating and trying interview situation, it is also a most rewarding and exciting learning experience.

The Paranoid/Hostile Patient

The final clinical syndrome to be addressed is the paranoid or hostile patient. Paranoid or hostile behaviors are found in a wide range of psychiatric disorders and in various degrees of severity. For purposes of this text those defenses common to the paranoid paient will be discussed. Primitive denial is present in all paranoids and is especially prominent in the overly delusional paranoid patient. The use of primitive denial is the individual's attempt to avoid awareness of the hurtful and painful aspects of reality. The paranoid patient often denies or disclaims any feelings toward a particular event or incident. The client is, in fact, overly sensitive to those traits in someone else that are denied in himself. The paranoid person also uses projection as a defense. Unable to accept or tolerate his own angry and volatile feelings, hostility and anger is projected on to others. He denies his own aggression and is insensitive to the impact of his behavior on others. The paranoid also uses the defense of reaction formation to keep from seeing his aggression, his needs for dependency and his warm, caring feelings. The client must, in fact, defend himself against his needs and characteristics and does so through the use of reaction formation.[2] The client is essentially saying that "if I don't care about you, then you cannot hurt or berate me."

These defenses generally are encountered early in the interview process. The patient will deny the existence of any problem or need for treatment or hospitalization.

The major characteristic of the paranoid encountered during the evaluation interview is anger. This anger may manifest itself through a number of different behaviors. The client might withdraw in an angry and silent manner or flood the interview in such a way as not to allow any discourse, refusing to see himself as a patient needing help. He is likely to mistrust the therapist and exhibit some hostility towards the interviewer. Finally, the paranoid patient might make demands upon the therapist which need to be addressed. These various behaviors need to be undersood and dealt with so as to establish some initial rapport.

Anger and silence may be best handled by acknowledging the patient's anger and by honestly stating the purpose and potential outcome of the interview.[2] For example, the patient may complain that he has told the story enough times and doesn't want to repeat it again. The therapist then needs to acknowledge the client's feelings and explain the reasons for this specific interview. Often, the paranoid or hostile patient, instead of being silent and sullen, will flood the interview wih a barrage of words. This flooding is actually the patient's attempt to dominate the interview. This need for dominance generally stems from the patient's feelings of worthlessness and inadequacy. In order to intercede, the interviewer may simply ask the patient how one may help him with his problems. In this way, the therapist will regain control of the interview and also show the patient that he, the therapist, will not be dominated. This stance is also a reassuring one to the patient.

With the paranoid patient, the therapist needs to maintain an honest, realistic and professional relationship, rather than a friendly, personal one. The paranoid patient's mistrust and hostility toward others is a central issue for this client. The paranoid patient both wishes for and fears closeness with others. The paranoid is unable to determine whom he can and cannot trust. This dilemma should be acknowledged and understood by the interviewer.

Finally, the paranoid and hostile patient is difficult for the beginning therapist. The challenge for the therapist is to come to grips with his own angry, hostile and aggressive impulses to grow both professionally and personally.

Essential Information for the Occupational Therapist

The occupational therapist is primarily concerned with how the individual relates to and functions within physical, psychologioal and social environments. The occupational therapist must assess the client's past and present level of functioning and the client's potenial for achieving a meaningful and functional life in the future. The areas of concern for psychiatric occupational therapy clients are the following:

1. Work/play history and current skills
2. Leisure time pursuits and interests
3. Daily living activities and time management
4. Mental status
5. Social history

Hemphill[4] states that obtaining the mental status examination and social history is not the responsibility of the occupational therapist. It is, however, information with which the occupational therapist must be familiar and must understand in terms of significance and relevance to the client's treatment.

Occupational therapy literature is replete with different types of evaluation tools and procedures fitting into various frames of reference and theoretical constructs. There have been some fruitful attempts to standardize evaluations since the early 1980s. Only through such efforts and results will the field of psychiatric occupational therapy continue to exist as a helping profession.

Work History/Play History

A client's current work skills and behavior are generally assessed through the use of task evaluations or simulated work situations. Within this volume, the Work Capacity Evaluation will be presented and discussed. This evaluation will primarily deal with the client's capacity to engage in the work process. It is often helpful to obtain a history of the client's work experiences. This history taking is best accomplished through the use of an extensive semi-structured interview. Such an instrument has been developed by Linda Moorhead.[5] The therapist must be familiar with the occupational behavior frame of reference and skilled in conducting a history-taking interview to be able to correctly use this procedure.

Just as an adult's work capacity and current level of functioning must be assessed, so must the child's ability to engage in play. The child's play history and current play experiences must be determined. Nancy Takata[10] has developed and described a play history evaluation. This play history is an open-ended questionnaire which attempts to identify play experiences and opportunities for the child. This history-taking interview, as well as Moorehead's interview, requires that the interviewer be able to ask questions and be able to elicit and clarify information pertinent to the areas under consideration.

Leisure Time Interests and Pursuits

The interests and activities of the client are often used by the occupational therapist as a primary medium for treatment. In order to obtain information regarding the person's past, current and potential interests, the occupational therapist often will use an interest checklist. This instrument was initially developed by Janice Matsutsuyu.[6] Adaptions to this instrument have been made and are widely used by practitioners. In the article, Ms. Matsutsuyu defines six propositions upon which the interest checklist and its subsequent analysis is based. The checklist is used in conjunction with a follow-up interview. This follow-up interview allows further exploration, elaboration and clarification of the information. Here again, the skills of the interviewer will determine to some extent the usefulness and completeness of the information obtained.

The occupational therapist, using this or any other evaluation tool or procedure, must be well-grounded in that particular frame of reference upon which the evaluation is based. To use a particular evaluation tool without this knowledge and without a rationale for its use, is both unproductive and unprofessional.

Daily Living Skills/Time Management

Occupational therapists are interested in how an individual occupies and manages time. The occupational therapist also is interesed in knowing the quality of the activity in which the individual is engaged. Numerous evaluations have been developed that assess the individual's ability to occupy and manage time. One such procedure was developed by Sandra Watanabe.[7] The activities configuration is of particular interest to the occupational therapist as it allows assessment of the specific activities in which the client engages, the function of these activities, their importance to the client and degree of competency. This interview procedure also can provide the client with a concrete picture of how he spends his time and what activities he does for himself or for others, either willingly or unwillingly. This kind of picture can sometimes be a starting point for treatment as it may become a barometer for change or a means of initiating self-reflection and self-evaluation in the client. The client and therapist may also use the tool to more accurately assess the client's current ability to manage his time, to problem-solve, and to use time more satisfactorily in the work, play and self-activities.

In addition to the activities configuration, the Barth Time Construction, which also assesses time management, has recently been described and is presented later in this book. It is a standardized evaluation used in a group format which assesses the quantity of time devoted to daily living, work, leisure activities and sleep.

Besides time management, the occupational therapist is concerned with the individual's ability to engage successfully in self-care activities or activities of daily living. Numerous evaluations have been developed which address this area of concern. Several procedures are presented in this book and will be described by their respective "developers." Each procedure is partially dependent upon the interviewing skills of the therapist for its success. These skills include the ability to listen, probe, observe, clarify or question in an effective and engaging manner.

While most occupational therapy evaluation procedures are semi-structured interviews, the BaFPE is standardized and structured. It is geared to obtaining information about the individual's functional performance and includes self-care activities. To maintain its validity and reliability, one needs to follow its directions of administration and interpretation.

Summary

This chapter defined interview and described briefly its purposes and essential components. An attempt was made to describe potential interview problems and how to interview difficult patients. This chapter also discussed the types of interviews that an occupational therapist might use and areas of focus or concern.

The interview is central to the helping process. It can be exciting, challenging and thrilling; it also demands a great deal of knowledge, skills and courage. To engage in the process of understanding and knowing another human being is difficult, tiring and potentially the most rewarding experience one human being can have with another being.

References
1. Sullivan HS (1954). The Psychiatric Interview. New York: Norton, 4.
2. MacKinnon R and Michaels R (1971). The Psychiatric Interview in Clinical Practice. Philadelphia: Saunders, 9, 194, 231, 246, 266, 278.
3. Reik T (1949). Listening With the Third Ear. New York: Grove Press, 144, 148.
4. Hemphill B (ed) (1983). The Evaluative Process in Psychiatric Occupational Therapy. Thorofare, New Jersey: Slack, 255.
5. Moorhead LM (1969). The occupational history. Am J Occup Ther 23, 329-334.
6. Matsutsuyu JS (1969). The interest checklist. Am J Occup Ther 23, 323-328.

7. Watanabe S (1968). Four concepts basic to occupational therapy process. Am J Occup Ther 22, 439-444.
8. Balinsky B and Burger R (1959). The Executive Interview—A Bridge to People. New York: Harper & Bros, 38.
9. Scott JC (1975). Influencing student observations. Am J Occup Ther 29, 143-145.
10. Takata N (1969). The play history. Am J Occup Ther 23, 314-318.

Bibliography

Argelander H (1976). The Initial Interview in Psychotherapy. New York: Human Sciences Press.

Benjamin A (1974). The Helping Interview (2nd ed). Boston: Houghton Mifflin.

Brill NI (1978). Working with People: The Helping Process (2nd ed). Philadelphia: Lippincott.

Davis JD (1971). The Interview as Arena. Stanford, California: Stanford University Press.

DeSchweinitz EK (1962). Interviewing in the Social Sciences. London, England: The National Council of Social Services.

Fenlason AF, Ferguson GB, and Abrahamson AC (1962). Essentials in Interviewing for the Interviewer Offering Professional Services. New York: Harper & Row.

Freedman A and Kaplan H (1967). Comprehensive Textbook of Psychiatry. Baltimore: Williams and Wilkins.

Garrett, A. (1972). Interviewing: Its Principles and Methods (2nd ed). New York: Family Service Association of America.

Gordon R (1975). Interviewing: Strategy, Techniques and tactics (revised ed). Homewood, Illinois: The Dorsey Press.

Hopkins HL and Smith HD (eds) (1978). Willard and Spackman's Occupational Therapy (5th ed). Philadelphia: Lippincott.

Kadushin A (1972). The Social Work Interview. New York: Columbia University Press.

Matarazzo JD and Wiens AN (1972). The Interview: Research on Its Anatomy and Structure. Chicago: Aldine Atherton.

Nemiah JC (1961). Foundations of Psychopathology. New York: Oxford University Press.

Okum BF (1976). Effective Helping: Interviewing and Counseling Techniques. North Scituate, Massachusetts: Duxburg Press.

Redlick FC and Freedman DX (1966). The Theory and Practice of Psychiatry. New York: Basic Books.

Richardson SA, Dohrenliend BS, and Klein D (1965). Interviewing: Its forms and functions. New York: Basic Books.

Stewart C and Cash W (1974). Interviewing: Principles and Practices. Dubuque, Iowa: Brown.

Woody RH and Woody JD (eds) (1972). Clinical Assessment in Counseling and Psychotherapy. Englewood Cliffs, New Jersey: Prentice-Hall.

CHAPTER 4

USE OF AN OCCUPATIONAL HISTORY INTERVIEW IN OCCUPATIONAL THERAPY

Gary Kiefhofner, Dr.PH, OTR, FAOTA
Alexis Henry, MS, OTR/L

Unlike the medical histories which appear in a familiar format in medical records everywhere, occupational therapy interviews are likely to vary in terms of how they are conducted, as well as how they are reported, and it is unlikely that one will find two therapists using the same format outside of the same hospital. Yet most therapists recognize the need for a thorough historical interview as the basis for understanding the patient's past and present state of functioning. Additionally, there is some agreement among therapists as to what areas should be explored in such a history. As a result, although the field lacks consensus as to the use of one particular historical interview, there have been several projects aimed at development of an occupational history interview. This chapter will trace the development of this type of history, from Moorhead's original Occupational History to the most recent addition of the Occupational Performance History Interview. It will examine general issues of reliability and validity with history interviews, as well as make specific recommendations for improving the reliability and validity of existing histories.

The Concept of a Historical Interview

Historical interviews have been used in other professions for both clinical and research purposes. As an approach to interviewing, a history may be used to understand the development of a person's beliefs and values, the formation of behavior, and the influence of socio-environmental forces on a person's lifestyle. In psychiatry, histories have frequently been used to elicit an account of the circumstances leading up to and interwoven with a particular emotional difficulty or series of emotional troubles.

In occupational therapy, histories have both overlapped with those used by other professionals and covered areas unique to occupational therapy. Typically, the occupational therapy interview may seek information about educational history, work experiences, leisure, activities of daily living, the use of time, and resources in the environment.

Moorhead, who developed the first published occupational history,[1] believed that the focus of this type of instrument should be to discover how a particular person was socialized into holding and performing certain occupational roles. Moorhead explicitly stated that the purpose of history-taking in occupational therapy was to understand the development of occupational behavior. As such, the author clearly placed the instrument within a theoretical framework unique to occupational therapy. Moorhead further argued that gathering a history represented the use of a particular scientific method. Within this perspective, the occupational history becomes the key to the occupational therapist's role as a research and clinical scientist.

Moorhead's Occupational History

Moorhead's semi-structured interview was designed to gather detailed qualitative information concerning functioning in various occupational roles. The author specified four basic foci to use in analyzing this data:

1. Learning and socialization in childhood roles
2. Exploration of the decision-making process around issues of occupational choice
3. Patterns of achievement and failure in occupations and environmental conditions which might influence these
4. Course of movement, and solidification or lack of it, in adult occupational roles.

Moorhead developed the instrument after an extensive review of literature pertaining to role theory, socialization, and occupational choice. Thus, the instrument appeared to be a valid expression of the chosen theoretical framework.

While Moorhead did not examine the reliability of the instrument, the author did conduct approximately 100 interviews with psychiatric clients. On the basis of these interviews, it was suggested that it would be possible to achieve a reliable interview since subjects found it non-threatening and relevant. To assist therapists with the interview and its interpretation, Moorhead developed a format for analyzing the intended result of each question.

Moorhead's Occupational History consisted of 76 suggested questions. As a result, one of the drawbacks to the instrument was that it could take well over an hour to conduct. Other possible deterrents to its use were that no means was provided for a concise narrative or quantitative summary, and that clinicians perceived it as being more appropriate for psychiatry than for physical dysfunction.

The Occupational Role History

Noting that the shift from long-term to acute care in psychiatry compelled therapists to use a briefer screening tool, Florey and

Michelman[2] developed and piloted the Occupational Role History. This instrument was based on Moorhead's work, and used an occupational behavior frame of reference. In addition, Florey and Michelman identified five critical areas about which the instrument is designed to provide information:

1. Sequence and continuity of occupational roles and their components

2. Ability of the subject to identify satisfaction and dissatisfaction with interests, people, tasks and the environment

3. The ability to perform and be comfortable in several occupational roles simultaneously

4. Areas of skills and deficit

5. Balance between work, chores and leisure

Florey and Michelman offer criteria for analyzing the results of the instrument, suggesting that two dimensions of behavior can be discerned from the interview. Role status, or the quality of performance over time, can be categorized as either functional, temporarily impaired or dysfunctional. The second dimension, balance, is a more qualitative judgment comparing the person's time spent in leisure with that spent in other occupational roles. Although Florey and Michelman do not describe the instrument's reliability, in the use of the instrument with 20 psychiatric patients, the authors found it capable of discriminating levels of occupational performance. It was also found that it filled a significant gap in patients' medical records, since patients' medical charts primarily related histories of symptomatology and family relationships without information on patients' occupational roles or skills.

The Occupational Role History in Physical Disabilities

Whereas the original occupational history was not intended solely for use in psychosocial dysfunction, Florey and Michelman's Occupational Role History was. Kielhofner, Harlan, Bauer, and Maurer[3] later modified this shorter history for use with physically disabled clients. The authors developed a rating scale which would allow for quantification of clinical judgments based on the interview. In this way, the authors were able to examine the types of clinical judgments that could be made as well as the reliability of the instrument. The rating scale used the model of human occupation as a theoretical framework; thus, it remained in the occupational behavior tradition used in the original occupational history and occupational role history.

The rating scale consists of 11 pairs of items, each designed to operationalize variables suggested by the theoretical model. Each item is rated on a scale of 1 to 5, from highly dysfunctional to highly functional behavior. The paired items together give a score for each model variable. Summed scores, representing the subsystems, the system and environment are also derived from the rating scale.

The authors administered the interview to 20 physically disabled men and women.[3] Each interview was audiotaped so that interrater reliability between two additional raters could be examined. Test-retest reliability was examined by retesting 10 of the 20 subjects. The interclass correlation coefficients for the two raters listening to each interview ranged from 0.93 to 0.38 on individual items; 18 of the 22 items achieved an acceptable level of reliability. The coefficient for the total summed scale was 0.85 (p = .0001) which, according to the authors, can be interpretted as "almost perfect agreement" for this statistic. Test-retest coefficients, averaged for the interviewer and two raters, ranged from a low of 0.59 to a high of 0.93 on individual items. Coefficients for the total score for each of the three raters were 0.93, 0.85, and 0.94 (p = .05). The study provided evidence of acceptable reliability of clinical judgments across interviews and raters when a systematic rating scale is used to reduce interview data into ratings and when the rating scale is based on a theoretical model with which the raters are familiar.

The Occupational Performance History Interview

The culmination of this evolution of history interviews is the Occupational Performance History Interview.[4] This instrument was developed in response to a decision by the American Occupational Therapy Association (AOTA) to fund a project that would lead to a standardized history which could be used by the profession. To meet this AOTA mandate, the final instrument was to be generic in nature (that is, applicable to therapists working with various types of patients and with different age groups), consistent with AOTA Uniform Terminology, valid and reliable.

Development of the instrument began with an extensive review of existing histories, both in occupational therapy and other fields.[4] Following this stage, a team of the project investigators and practicing therapists identified and defined five major content areas to be the basis of the interview. These content areas and definitions were submitted to a panel of occupational therapy experts before the first draft of the history was written.

The next stage of development consisted of a field test of the first questionnaire version, a rating scale for quantifying the obtained historical information, and a manual describing how to use the instrument and scale. Approximately 90 therapists used and critiqued the interview materials. The final research version of the Occupational Performance History Interview consisted of 39 recommended questions covering the five content areas. The content areas were chosen to provide a holistic picture of the client's functioning in the everyday performance of occupational behavior. These areas were environmental influences, life roles, organization of daily living routines, perceptions of ability and responsibility, and interests, values and goals.

The area of environmental influences is explored by questions pertaining to human and non-human resources and barriers in the subject's past, present and anticipated environments, and the extent to which they have influenced the subject's adaptation. In the area of life roles, the interviewer examines the client's pattern of role involvement and performance in these roles. Organization of daily living routines includes questions about the subject's typical use of time, the adaptiveness of time-use patterns, and the person's balance of work, play and self-care tasks. Perceptions of ability and responsibility concern the subject's awareness of and willingness to take responsibility for life decisions. In addition, the interviewer attempts to determine the degree to which the subject's perceptions of ability are realistic. Finally, the area of interests, values and goals refers to the person's ability to identify and act on personal values, interests and goals, and to attain satisfaction from them.

In addition to the semi-structured interview format, a rating scale was developed to quantify the subject's functioning in each of the five content areas in both the past and the present. The rating scale consists of two items for each of the five areas. Each item is rated twice, once for the past and once for the present, on a scale of 1 to 5, with 5 being completely adaptive and 1 being completely maladaptive. Eight of the 10 items refer to the individual's behavior and two refer to the environment.

Reliability Studies

This instrument was subjected to an examination of test-retest and interrater reliability.[4] The instrument was administered to a total of 153 subjects by teams of therapists. The first interview with each patient was audiotaped. Between 5 and 12 days later, each patient was re-interviewed by the partner of the therapist who had conducted the first interview. The original audiotapes were duplicated and sent to two additional therapists who rated the interview. Interrater reliability data were obtained in this fashion for 129 of the original subjects. A total of 201 therapists participated in either administering the interviews or rating the tapes.

Patients represented a spectrum of psychiatric and physical disabilities, and ranged in age from 13 to 93. Therapists had an average of seven years in practice, a wide variety of experience with interviews, and were most likely to identify with an eclectic frame of reference.

Item-total correlations on the rating scale were moderately high, and correlations between past and present ratings were generally low, indicating that the scale was relatively homogeneous, and that judgments of past and present behavior could be made independently. Test-retest correlation coefficients for ratings of present behavior ranged from 0.31 to 0.49 on individual items and were 0.35 for the environmental subtotal, 0.54 for the individual subtotal and 0.53 for the scale total. For ratings of past behavior, coefficients ranged from 0.55 to 0.68, with 0.63 for the environmental subscale and 0.73 for the individual subscale and for the total scale. Overall, the test-retest coefficients appeared lower for the psychiatric patients than for geriatric and physically disabled groups.

While the ratings of past behavior generally showed acceptability over time, those of the present did not. There were several possible reasons for this. First, a large number of therapists participated in the collection of data, and the conditions during the first and second interviews were not identical. Another major source of error was that therapists did not always use the same point in the patient's life to demarcate past and present. Obviously, this judgment was easier to make with physically disabled patients, when the present might be indicated by a traumatic injury or the clear onset of an illness.

Interrater reliability coefficients ranged from 0.38 to 0.55 on past items and from -0.08 to 0.46 on present items. For the environmental subscale, individual subscale, and the scale total, coefficients were 0.57, 0.60, and 0.63 respectively for past ratings and 0.13, 0.50, and 0.48 respectively for present ratings. While this level of stability does not meet acceptable criteria, it is important to realize that interrater reliability in this study was somewhat unusual in that the same two raters were not compared throughout. Thus, the opportunity for two raters to become increasingly familiar with an instrument over time did not exist.

An interesting factor observed during analysis was that when therapists shared a frame of reference, their ratings of the interviews were more likely to agree. The importance of this point for achieving a reliable history will be considered later in this chapter.

Discussion

The State of the Art of History Taking

The use of an occupational history of some sort is widespread, although many clinicians rely on their own version rather than on one of the existing published instruments. However, recognition in the profession of the need for a standardized approach to history taking is creating an impetus for change. The question, then, is whether any of the existing histories can fill the role of being a standardized instrument for the field as a whole.

To answer this question does not need to suggest that therapists use only one occupational history and no other history or interview. It will always be necessary to have specialized histories to allow the therapist to explore some facet of patient functioning in fuller detail, for example, a leisure history or work history. Further, the history does not take the place of a functional assessment or assessments. What it should do, however, is provide a common base or frame for conceptualizing patients' lives and understanding the impact of stress, illness or trauma on patients' lives. Having this common frame implies that there are areas of patients' lives that all occupational therapists are interested in, regardless of the patient's age or diagnosis, and it communicates to other professionals that they can expect to find certain areas of content when they read the occupational therapist's records.

Of the existing published histories, perhaps Moorhead's Occupational History has achieved the widest recognition. It appears to be the earliest published approach to history taking in the field, and it is taught in many psychosocial occupational therapy classes. At the same time, it appears to be less frequently used in the area of physical dysfunction.

Compared to the other histories discussed in this chapter, the Occupational Performance History Interview is the only one that strives to be as comprehensive as the Occupational History. However, its structure deviates markedly from Moorhead's instrument. The latter is organized around performance in specific roles, i.e., student, homemaker or worker, and leisure.

With the Occupational Performance History Interview, life roles comprise just one of five content areas. As a result, there is a more explicit focus on variables that affect performance in life roles—that is, interest, values, goals, personal responsibility— and more depth is given to the area of environmental influences.

An important difference between the Occupational Performance History Interview and the Occupational History is the addition of a rating scale to the Occupational Performance History Interview. The rating scale makes it possible to examine reliability as well as to use the instrument as a predictive or concurrent measure in research. Unfortunately, while nothing is known about the reliability of the Occupational History, what is known about the reliability of the Occupational Performance History Interview suggests that further development is needed. (A second study of reliability of the Occupational Performance History Interview, funded by AOTA/AOTF, is underway). There is reason to believe that the reliability of this instrument can be improved in studies and that there are factors which a therapist can consider and use to maximize the effectiveness of a history interview as a clinical assessment.

Improving the Reliability of Historical Interviews

In the study of the reliability of a historical interview by Kielhofner, et al.,[3] acceptably high coefficients were generally obtained. One difference between this study of the Occupational Role History in physical disabilities and that of the Occupational Performance History Interview study was that the Occupational Role History used only three raters, and all were trained in the use of the instrument and rating scale. Many of the raters in the Occupational Performance History Interview study had never used any form of interview before, and all received training for the instrument from a written manual. Therefore, the low reliability coefficients obtained in the study of the Occupational Performance History Interview may reflect not just inexperience with interviews, but also problems in the manual itself or in learning an interview process through self-study. Even more significant, perhaps, is that the Occupational Role History rating scale was explicitly based on a theoretical frame of reference with which the raters were familiar. While the Occupational Performance History Interview reflected some general theoretical assumptions about occupational behavior, it was not designed to represent any one frame of reference. However, the reliability of this instrument was higher among therapists holding the same frame of reference, and it was higher for therapists adhering to an occupational behavior frame of reference.[4]

The implication is that one way to achieve a reliable interview may be to base the interview and rating scale on a specific frame of reference. Clinicians using the interview would then need to be knowledgeable of the concepts and tenets upon which it is based. This is not an unreasonable expectation, however. Certainly, many instruments, in both occupational therapy and other fields, require the user to demonstrate familiarity with the principles underlying the instrument's development, as well as with the skills required to use it. Although not a history, the Southern California Sensory Integrative Tests are an example of a battery for which the user must be trained and demonstrate proficiency.

Basing an instrument on a frame of reference does not mean that all clinicians must hold that frame of reference. What it does mean is that clinicians who use the instrument must have sufficient understanding of it and must use it in ways that are compatible with its theoretical framework. This, in turn, means that clinical reasoning or problem-solving proceeds from a carefully thought-out plan of action in which the therapist chooses assessments because he wants to be able to conceptualize the patient's problems in a particular way and knows that the chosen instruments will allow him to do so.

Obviously, reliability does not come solely from the consistent use of a frame of reference with a given history. Especially with an instrument such as the Occupational Performance History Interview, certain definitions and criteria for administration and rating are necessary. If the history is to provide a rating of both past and present behavior, then raters must be able to agree on the demarcation between past and present, even when no immediately recognizable marker exists. Therapists may also need to balance the interview with background demographic information before completing the ratings. Finally, with a semi-structured interview, therapists must realize that the provided questions are intended only as a guide, not as a limit. If other questions are needed or are more appropriate to a given patient's circumstances, then the therapist should be prepared to deviate from the provided format.

Future Directions

Interestingly, apart from research related to developing occupational histories, there is little indication that histories have been used in studies of predictive, concurrent, or discriminative validity. While the existing occupational histories all appear to have content and face validity, the authors have only anecdotal evidence to suggest that the information obtained from such a history can be used accurately to make predictions about patients' future performances. Further, there is little more than hypothetical support for the notion that there would be a relationship between a patient's reported historical ways of performing and what might be observed on a functional assessment. This is the kind of information that will make an occupational history a truly vital part of clinical practice.

At present, therapists seem more likely to use histories as a means of establishing rapport than as a key to future treatment directions. This is unfortunate because the history can be a rich source of clinical information. It may, however, be the role of research to point the way. Therefore, an important future direction in the development of the occupational history will be to examine its place in clinical decision making. For example, questions that might be explored include the following: Are there identifiable historical patterns that relate to diagnostic groups; to functional status? Can the history be used to identify an appropriate level of treatment for a patient? Can the history be used for prognostic and pre-discharge planning decisions?

Summary

While further development of occupational histories obviously is required, it remains for the therapist to make optimal use of existing instruments. Adhering to some simple guidelines can enhance the properties of any history. First, the therapist should make an attempt to select and use an appropriate existing historical interview and to become familiar with the instrument, its properties and limitations, and the author's intent for its use. The therapist should also make a conscious effort to employ a frame of reference for interpretation of the data. While the therapist may use another compatible frame of reference for overall assessment and treatment, an instrument with a specified frame of reference should be applied accordingly. The therapist should also be aware of and seek to control factors which affect respondent consistency, honesty and thoroughness in responding to questions. These include rapport with the patient, information the patient has about how the interview data will be used, adequate preparation of the patient for the interview and therapist sensitivity to feelings and perceptions on the part of the patient which might influence responses to questions. Additional factors which affect the stability and accuracy of an interview are generally noted by the interview's author. By being aware of an interview's nature and properties, and by carefully using the history interview, the clinician can conduct an effective and optimal assessment.

References
1. Moorhead LC (1969). The occupational history. Am J Occup Ther 23, 329-334.
2. Florey LL and Michelman SM (1982). Occupational role history: A screening tool for psychiatric occupational therapy. Am J Occup Ther 36, 301-308.
3. Kielhofner G, Harlan B, Bauer D, and Maurer P (1986). The reliability of a historical interview with physically disabled respondents. Am J Occup Ther 40, 551-556.
submitted for review).
4. Kielhofner G and Henry AD: Development and Investigation of an Occupational Performance History Interview. Am J Occup Ther, in press.

CHAPTER 5

THE ROLE CHECKLIST

Roann Barris, EdD, OTR
Frances Oakley, MS, OTR
Gary Kielhofner, DrPH, OTR

The Role Checklist was developed by Oakley[1] to operationalize a construct within the model of human occupation.[2,3] This construct, roles, has been integral not only to the occupational behavior tradition, but also to a variety of other models or frames of reference in occupational therapy.[4] This chapter will begin with an overview of the concept of role as it pertains to occupational therapy in general, and to the model of human occupation in particular, followed by a discussion of previous approaches that have been used to collect data on roles.

Roles

Role is a sociological concept that has its origins in theater.[5,6] A role refers to a set of activities or behaviors that are engaged in by a person in a particular situation, as prescribed by that situation.[5] The set of behaviors that make up a certain role have a degree of consistency or recognizability that is inherent in the role, and not in the particular individual performing or occupying the role. Because of this attribute, the role serves to organize a person's behavior—that is, the role provides guidelines to the individual about appropriate ways to dress, forms of interacting with other individuals, tasks to perform, and uses of time.[7] As a result, roles become not only the framework for carrying out daily life, but also the means to achieving competency in daily life.[6]

Occupational therapy, in its concern for competent performance of life tasks, has found the concept of role to be useful in understanding and recognizing both functional and dysfunctional behavior.[8] Reilly[9] was one of the earliest theorists in occupational therapy to emphasize the relevance of this concept.[4,10] In a description of the professional curriculum at the University of Southern California, Reilly proposed that the concept of role was one of the critical parameters in the theoretical framework for occupational therapy practice.[9] Reilly suggested that social psychology had distinguished three subsystems of roles—gender identification roles, group membership roles, and occupational roles—and that the latter should be the domain of occupational therapy interest. The definition of occupational roles included preschooler (because play was considered the "work" of the child), student, worker, housewife, and retiree. Until fairly recently this conceptualization of occupational roles generally was accepted by other theorists in the field and influenced the focus of instruments designed to assess role performance.

Whereas initial interest in roles focused on the process of acquiring and changing roles throughout one's lifespan,[6,10] later exploration of this concept focused more on identifying the ways in which roles become organizing frameworks for daily life. In the model of human occupation,[2,3] the role is a major component of the habituation subsystem, which is responsible for the organization and performance of routine behavior. The model outlines three dimensions of roles: perceived incumbency, internalized expectations, and role balance.[3] Perceived incumbency refers to an individual's belief that one occupies a role. Internalized expectations are the behaviors recognized by a person as comprising role performance; thus, two people occupying the same role in title may differ in terms of the demands or obligations which are associated with that role. Role balance refers to the capacity to maintain harmony among roles,[2,3] both daily and over time.

All three dimensions of roles influence the total system's organization. Thus, too few or too many roles in one's life, unawareness or misconceptions regarding performance expectations for a role, conflicts between role demands, or an imbalance in time allotted to roles can result in maladaptive occupational performance. Similarly, not replacing lost roles at times of transition can be problematic.

Another recent change in the use of roles in occupational therapy was the recognition that the original delineation of occupational roles was incomplete for identifying all roles in which people engage in work, play, and self-maintenance activities. For example, family group-membership roles, such as parent and spouse, organize not ony sexual and social behaviors, but occupational behavior as well. That is, family roles shape and require certain forms of leisure, self-care, and work. In addition, the original typology of roles subordinated the role of player in adulthood to the role of worker,[9] suggesting that adult leisure is only a secondary concern. Apart from the dubious nature of such an assertion, roles such as volunteer, hobbyist, or amateur may be important sources of achievement and intrinsic satisfaction for adults who are unable either to work at paying jobs or to find sufficient satisfaction in their work. Further, the role of retiree does not indicate how one uses one's time; instead, it describes an economic status. Therefore, it follows that a role should be considered to have occupational components (and thus be of concern to occupational therapists) if it provides opportunities for the performance of productive or play-ful activity.[1,3]

Assessment of Roles

Several approaches to gathering data on roles have been developed by occupational therapists. These approaches primarily employ interviews of varying lengths and yield qualitative data which may then be supplemented by data from other, more objective, assessments.

The Occupational History is perhaps the most well-known of these interviews.[11] This interview includes extensive questions about the subject's socialization to and performance in the roles of worker, student, housewife, and family member. The interview attempts to identify key influences or role models for the subject, problems and strengths in the performance of each role, sources of satisfaction and dissatisfaction with each, and environmental supports and constraints to performance. As with other history interviews, the Occupational History cannot be quantified. Thus, while it is a potentially rich source of qualitative information, little is known about its reliability or validity.

The Occupational Role History,[12] a modification of the Occupational History, was developed to provide a shorter interview that could be used as a screening assessment with patients. A rating scale was subsequently developed to provide a quantitative evaluation of the information elicited by the interview.[13] This approach has the advantage of yielding both qualitative and quantitative data, and is somewhat less time-consuming than the original Occupational History.

While several other interview formats exist (for example, the Adolescent Role Assessment[14] and the Environmental Questionnaire[15]), occupational therapists nevertheless have continued to lack an efficient means for assessing the extent to which a person actually identifies with a particular role and values the role. The Role Checklist is an instrument whose conceptual roots lie in occupational behavior and the model of human occupation. It assesses the individual's perception of participation in roles with occupational components throughout the lifespan, provides information regarding an individual's capacity to maintain continuity in and a balance among roles, and indicates the degree to which each role is valued. Because this is a written checklist, the instrument is easily and quickly completed.

The Role Checklist: Description, Administration, and Development

Description of Instrument

The Role Checklist (Appendix A and B) is a written inventory that is appropriate for use with adolescents, adults, and elderly persons with physical or psychosocial dysfunction. The instrument is divided into two parts.

Part One assesses, along a temporal continuum, the major roles that serve to organize a person's life. Ten roles are included in the instrument: student, worker, volunteer, care giver, home maintainer, friend, family member, religious participant, hobbyist/amateur, and participant in organizations. Each role is defined in terms of its occupational components—for example, friend is defined as "spending time or doing something, at least once a week, with a friend." In addition to these 10 roles, a space for "other" is included. The roles are presented in a grid consisting of three columns labeled "past," "present," and "future," and individuals are instructed to check those columns that apply to their performance of each role.

Part Two of the Role Checklist measures the degree to which the individual values each role. The roles are repeated under the headings "not at all valuable," "somewhat valuable," and "very valuable." Individuals are instructed to check the column that best describes the value they attribute to each role, even if they have not performed or do not anticipate performing the role.

Administration

The following set of directions has been developed to standardize administration of the Role Checklist:

Instruct individuals to complete the demographic information at the top of the checklist.

Part One. (1) Ask the client to read the instructions.

(2) Inquire if the instructions are understood and answer any questions pertaining to the administration of Part One.

(3) Define the time frame as follows: "The present refers not only to today, but also includes the previous seven days. Past refers to the period of time up until seven days ago. Future is anytime from tomorrow onward."

Part Two. (1) When individuals have completed Part One, ask the client to read the instructions for Part Two.

(2) Inquire if the instructions are understood and answer any questions pertaining to the administration of Part Two.

(3) Define valuable as follows: "Valuable refers to the worth you place on each role—that is, how important or desirable the role is to you." Remain with them until the checklist is completed.

Development and Content Validity

A review of social psychology, sociology, and occupational therapy literature revealed more than 20 roles related to family, work, and leisure activities. Some of these roles elaborated similar types of relationships, for example, aunt or cousin, while others clearly prescribed uses of time. The major criterion for inclusion of a particular role in the first version of the instrument was that it contain implications for productive time use. Thus, roles such as cousin or aunt were included under the more generic heading of family member.

Some traditional occupational therapy roles were excluded from the list. The role of homemaker was not included as such, but was divided into two roles believed to represent distinct forms of occupational behavior—home maintainer and care giver. These two roles appear to be non-gender-specific, as opposed to the role of homemaker, which has strong gender associations for many people. The role of retiree was also excluded from the instrument on the assumption that the status of retirement does not indicate how one's daily life is organized.

A preliminary list of roles was submitted to graduate students, faculty, and therapists for review. Their feedback supported the content validity of the proposed role taxonomy and pointed to the need to define each role in terms of occupational and frequency criteria. For example, the role of family member was defined as spending time or doing something *at least once a week* with another family member, such as a spouse, child, parent, or other relative. The importance of the frequency criterion in this role is that people may view themselves as family members, but their family may reside out of town, resulting in infrequent contact. Consequently, that role is not available to organize present daily life.

Early feedback further indicated that the role of leisure participant could actually be separated into three distinct roles: hobbyist/amateur, religious participant, and participant in organizations. Although all three address avocational pursuits, the direction of these pursuits is different for each, and each may be important in a person's life. Subsequent discussion of the role of religious participant also suggested that the spiritual act of worshipping should not be included in the definition of that role. Although worship is interrelated with occupational behavior—for example, getting dressed to go to church—worship itself is a spiritual activity. Religious participant was thus defined in the final version of the instrument as "Involvement, at least once a week, in groups or activities affiliated with one's religion (excluding worship)."

Pilot Testing

A version of the instrument with 10 roles was used in a pilot study for clarity and reliability with 17 undergraduate occupational therapy students. Respondents were asked to indicate what roles were occupied in the past and present, and their future intent to occupy roles. Median percent agreement on two administrations of the instrument, two weeks apart, was 82%. This version of the instrument was also field tested for clinical utility and relevance with an inpatient psychiatric population.[1] Clinical use led to refinements of the role definitions and also revealed an inadequacy in the first version of the instrument. That is, it was insufficient for a therapist to learn solely about perceived role incumbency, because people attach different values to performing different roles. A relevant question for therapy is whether or not an individual is performing valued roles. Thus, Part Two of the instrument, which asks about personal valuation for each role, was added to the checklist.

Reliability

The Role Checklist was administered by graduate occupational therapy students to 124 normal adults on two separate occasions. This group consisted primarily of white, female, well-educated subjects. Approximately half were between the ages of 18 and 30, and half between 31 and 65. Fifty percent of the subjects were married.

Kappa and percent agreement were computed to examine test-retest reliability in the population of 124 subjects and in subgroups defined by age and amount of time between test administrations. Both kappa and percent agreement were used because each has desirable properties. Percent agreement is a widely used and familiar statistic that is more readily understandable than kappa. However, it is limited as an estimate of reliability since it does not account for chance agreement. Kappa is a measure of agreement which corrects for chance; however, when observed agreement is close to perfect, kappa may actually be low since its calculation is based in part on the variability in responses.[16] It is therefore useful to compare kappa with percent agreement.

Table 5-1
Guidelines for Interpretation of Kappa

Kappa Statistic	Strength of Agreement
<0.00	Poor
0.00 - 0.20	Slight
0.21 - 0.40	Fair
0.41 - 0.60	Moderate
0.61 - 0.80	Substantial
0.81 - 1.00	Almost Perfect

The estimate of kappa for each role was a weighted average of each of the estimates of kappa for the categories of past, present, and future. In addition, a weighted estimate of kappa for each of the roles was obtained. Guidelines developed by Landis and Koch[17] for interpreting the kappa statistic appear in Table 5-1.

Table 5-2 presents estimates of kappa, weighted kappa, and percent agreement for Part One of the Role Checklist for the 124 subjects. The matrix of estimates for each role at the time points provides a description of each component. It is not provided as a basis for selecting the best subset of roles or time references; the major intent of this research was to evaluate the test instrument as a single entity.

Estimates of kappa for individual roles for a given time point ranged from slight to almost perfect agreement with the majority either moderate or substantial. Percent agreement for these components ranged from 73% to 97%, with the majority exceeding 88%.

Estimates of weighted kappa for each role over the three time points ranged from moderate to substantial with the majority falling in the substantial category. Percent agreement for each role ranged from 77% to 93%, with an average of 87%.

The estimates of weighted kappa for each time point over the 10 roles were substantial for the present, while estimates for the past and future were moderate. Percent agreement averaged 87%, with little appreciable difference noted among the time points. The estimates of weighted kappa for all roles for Part One of the test indicated substantial concordance; the composite estimate of percent agreement was 87%.

The effects of age of the subject and of time between test administrations were of interest. Table 5-3 presents estimates of weighted kappa and percent agreement for each role for two age groups and also for two time intervals for Part One of the Role Checklist.

Table 5-2
Kappa, Weighted Kappa, and Percent Agreement for the Role Checklist, Part One. (Perceived Incumbency)

	TIME CATEGORIES						OVERALL ROLE	
	Past		Present		Future			
ROLE	K	Percent Agreement	K	Percent Agreement	K	Percent Agreement	Wgtd K	Percent Agreement
Student	.55	95	.87	94	.65	84	.79	91
Worker	.32	85	.83	96	.40	87	.64	89
Volunteer	.43	79	.49	82	.49	76	.48	79
Care Giver	.56	81	.71	85	.71	90	.67	85
Home Maintainer	.51	91	.65	97	.20	90	.45	93
Friend	.42	90	.49	90	.40	89	.44	90
Family Member	.64	94	.78	91	.60	92	.72	92
Religious Participant[1]	.58	89	.77	89	.76	89	.74	89
Hobbyist/ Amateur	.40	89	.71	88	.49	90	.61	90
Participant in Organizations	.57	81	.36	76	.47	73	.48	77
Overall Time Categories Weighted K	.51		.74		.59			
Percent Agreement		87		89		86		

[1]Note: Data collected on previous version.

Almost all of the estimates of weighted kappa for age and time of testing were either moderate or substantial, with percent agreement ranging from 73% to 95%. Negative estimates of weighted kappa were obtained for a few roles. While unusual, such values are valid and reflect the method used to calculate kappa. For example, these values occurred when all subjects checked only one response during either the first or second administration of the checklist. In other words, these values of kappa may reflect a low variability in responses. In general, there was a tendency for the measures of concordance to be stronger for the older adults (31 to 79 years of age) than for the younger subgroup (18 to 30 years) and for the

Table 5-3
Weighted Kappa and Percent Agreement for Each Role by Age and Time of Testing Role Checklist, Part One. (Perceived Incumbency)

	OVERALL TIME CATEGORIES							
	AGE				WEEKS			
	18-30 N=64		31-79 N=60		1-4 N=87		7-5 N=37	
ROLE	Wgtd K	Percent Agreement	Wgtd K	Percent Agreement	Wgtd K	Percent Agreement	Wgtd K	Percent Agreement
Student	.78	92	.72	90	.80	91	.77	91
Worker	.73	91	.43	88	.88	94	−.10	79
Volunteer	.43	78	.53	81	.50	80	.43	76
Care Giver	.42	82	.77	89	.67	86	.66	85
Home Maintainer	.44	91	.45	95	.48	92	.79	95
Friend	−.05	89	.57	89	.50	92	.37	86
Family Member	.66	91	.77	94	.76	94	.61	90
Religious Participant[1]	.77	90	.72	87	.79	90	.65	85
Hobbyist/ Amateur	.61	88	.61	89	.65	91	.54	83
Participant in Organi- zations	.37	73	.81	89	.44	76	.57	79
Overall Roles								
Weighted K	.34		.70		.71		.43	
Percent Agreement		79		89		89		85

[1]Note: Data collected on previous version.

early retesting (one to four weeks), as opposed to later retesting (five to eight weeks).

Table 5-4 presents estimates of kappa, weighted kappa, and percent agreement for the value components for the 124 subjects. The weighted estimate of kappa over all roles indicated moderate concordance; the composite estimate of percent agreement was 79%. As before, estimates for subgroups classified by age and by time of testing were also obtained. Strength of agreement was most often moderate or above, with percent agreement usually exceeding 76%. Again, older subjects appeared to be more consistent in

Table 5-4
Kappa, Weighted Kappa, and Percent Agreement for the Total Group and for Age and Time of Testing
Role Checklist, Part Two. (Value)

ROLE	Total Sample N=124		AGE 18-30 N=64		AGE 31-79 N=60		WEEKS 1-4 N=87		WEEKS 5-8 N=37	
	K	Percent Agreement	K	Percent Agreement	K	Percent Agreement	K	Percent Agreement	K	Percent Agreement
Student	.65	87	.62	88	.65	84	.66	89	.60	81
Worker	.37	87	.25	86	.49	86	.39	86	.40	86
Volunteer	.48	73	.43	68	.51	73	.47	70	.51	74
Care Giver	.43	78	.44	77	.40	77	.42	75	.41	82
Home Maintainer	.55	76	.52	73	.58	77	.58	76	.48	72
Friend	.50	86	.27	86	.57	83	.49	86	.46	80
Family Member	.25	88	.11	85	.48	90	.32	88	.22	85
Religious Participant[1]	.67	79	.60	73	.73	82	.67	78	.60	74
Hobbyist/ Amateur	.42	72	.49	74	.35	67	.52	76	.17	58
Participant in Organizations	.27	64	.33	65	.21	60	.40	70	-.02	45
Overall Roles										
Percent Weighted K	.50		.44		.53		.53		.37	
Percent Agreement		79		78		78		79		74

[1]Note: Data collected on previous version.

their responses than younger subjects, and the association decreased with increasing retest intervals.

The assessment of the value of roles appeared less consistent than the assessment of perceived incumbency of roles. This may reflect how the data were measured. Three responses were possible for measuring values, whereas the measure of perceived incumbency was binary. Measures of agreement tend to decrease as the number of possible outcomes increase.

The version of the Role Checklist used for examining reliability contained an earlier wording of the definition for religious participant. Therefore, one cannot assume that the reliability of this item, which would affect the overall instrument reliability, would be the same in the current version. However, the authors do not anticipate an appreciable difference in the reliability of the total checklist.

This initial study of the Role Checklist's reliability suggests that the instrument is reasonably stable over time with normal adult subjects. Whether or not similar reliability would be obtained with various patient populations is not currently known. However, the instrument has been used clinically and in research; some examples will be described in the next section.

Research Using the Role Checklist

The Role Checklist has been used as part of a battery of assessments in several studies designed to compare groups of subjects. In one, data were collected on two groups of adolescents—adolescents who were hospitalized for psychosocial problems and non-hospitalized high school students.[18] Part Two of the Role Checklist was used as a measure of values and Part One as a measure of perceived incumbency in roles. In terms of perceived incumbency, the groups differed only in the number of present roles, no doubt reflecting the disruption caused by hospitalization. However, a trend appeared among non-hospitalized subjects toward planning to assume more roles in the future, while no such trend emerged in the hospitalized adolescents. On Part Two of the instrument, a significant difference in the valuation given to roles was found between the two groups, with the non-hospitalized subjects attaching more overall value to roles than did the hospitalized group. In addition, there was a tendency for the hospitalized adolescents to attribute less value to the roles of student, care giver, and organization participant than did the non-hospitalized subjects.

In another study of adolescents, subjects with medical-psychiatric diagnoses, subjects with psychiatric diagnoses only, and normal subjects were compared.[19] Although differences among the groups were slight, the number of non-valued roles was a key variable in a discriminant analysis model. Again, a greater tendency to value roles was associated with normal subjects.

The Role Checklist also has been used in research with elderly populations. One study examined the relationship between the amount of activity offered in three nursing homes, and residents' future orientation and present internalization of roles.[20] The number of future roles identified in the Role Checklist was used as one measure of future orientation, and the number of present roles was used to operationalize present role internalization. Activity availability showed a significant correlation with both these variables, suggesting that the presence of activity in the environment can have a positive effect on individuals' perceptions of themselves as active, occupational beings.

Finally, a study of non-institutionalized elderly subjects hypothesized that individuals performing a greater number of occupational roles would be more likely to experience greater life satisfaction.[21] This hypothesis was supported by the research, thereby providing some empirical evidence for the belief that involvement in occupational roles can contribute to the maintenance or restoration of adaptive behavior.

Clinical Use of the Role Checklist

The Role Checklist can be used with individuals ranging in age from adolescence to older adulthood, and it is not specific to a type of disability. Patients with both physical and psychosocial disabilities are likely to experience role changes; these changes may both result from disability and contribute to further disability. For example, the disruption in performance of the family or worker role during hospitalization can lead to a loss of relevant skills and a weakening of social ties, making re-entry into these roles at a later date exceedingly difficult.[22,23] In psychosocial practice, the patient who has been hospitalized several times for severe mental illness may experience a great deal of discontinuity in role performance to the extent that he may no longer perceive himself as occupying any role.[1] Rolelessness has, in fact, been identified as a critical problem with the young adult chronic patient.[24]

Apart from the discontinuity of role performance, several other key problem areas related to role incumbency can be identified by this instrument. In some cases the loss of a valued role—for example, giving up the worker role upon retirement—may be an integral component of the person's psychosocial disorder. In others, an individual may perceive him in too many roles and be unable to cope with the demands created by each. Some people may identify themselves as filling certain roles that are not meaningful or valuable to him and be frustrated at expending energy in directions that are not leading to attainment of his goals. The following case example describes an adult male who lacks an adequate number of present roles to organize his daily life and who is not fulfilling valued roles.

Case Study

Martin was a 46-year-old divorced white male with a history of recurring depression. He had been hospitalized on several occasions in the previous 20 years and received various somatic treatments as well as psychotherapy. Presently, he was not hospitalized, but was experiencing difficulties in his daily life, and was referred to an occupational therapist in private practice. The Role Checklist was administered as part of an initial battery, which also included the Occupational History,[11] the Interest Checklist,[25,26] and the Occupational Questionnaire.[27]

Martin came from a small town in a predominantly rural state. He described himself as being a bright child and a good student, and recalled that his family life was pleasant. As a high school student he was equipment manager for one of the teams, and was very involved in dramatics. In talking about his childhood, Martin was unable to remember any vocational fantasies and did not identify his father as a role model, although there were considerable parallels between his father's work history and his own. His father held a series of jobs before eventually settling into a low-level government position; a standing joke in the family concerned his father's inability to get along with employers.

Martin began college intending to major in languages or international affairs. Younger than his peers, he did not do well in his classes, was blackballed from a fraternity, and spent much of his time drinking, gambling, and engaging in other unproductive forms of leisure. After his sophomore year he married and did not return to college. He had two children.

For the past 20 years or so, Martin worked in various sales jobs. In his most recent, he was employed by a friend and was trying to sell hearing aids. Martin described a pattern of initial enthusiasm about a job, throwing himself into the work, and then losing interest.

Table 5-5
Results of Role Checklist. (Martin)

Role	Past	Present	Future	Not Valuable	Somewhat Valuable	Very Valuable
Student	X			X		
Worker	X	X	X			X
Volunteer				X		
Care Giver	X		X			X
Home Maintainer	X	X	X			X
Friend						X
Family Member	X	X	X			X
Religious Participant	X		X		X	
Hobbyist/ Amateur	X		X		X	
Participant in Organizations				X		

Problems at work tended to arise around interpersonal relationships, keeping detailed records, and having too much responsibility. While he disliked structure and rules, he nevertheless felt that he took advantage of unstructured situations.

Martin described a lack of close friends, although he did have a current relationship with a woman. His present life style was somewhat unstructured despite his job, and he pursued relatively few leisure interests. He also had very limited financial resources.

Following the interview, Martin completed the written instruments. The results of the Role Checklist are presented in Table 5-5. This instrument graphically showed both the therapist and Martin several noteworthy facts about the organization of his daily life and contradictions between his goals and current life style.

Martin identified only three continuous roles—worker, home maintainer, and family member—although he was not hospitalized at the time and could potentially have been enacting other roles. In fact, there were six roles which he rated as being very valuable to him; yet, he was filling only three of these. He considered the role of friend very valuable, but did not identify it as a future role. He had no actual plans for beginning to perform the three roles that he had identified for the future (caregiver, religious participant, and hobbyist/amateur).

Following discussion of the assessment results, Martin and the therapist developed a concrete plan of action which directly related to performance of valued roles. For example, Martin had indicated a strong interest in cooking. It was apparent that this interest could be readily incorporated into both the amateur role and the friendship role if Martin and his girlfriend invited friends over for a dinner. Cooking could also potentially reactivate the student role for Martin if he explored the possibility of taking cooking and catering courses at the local community college. Martin also realized that he wanted to make plans to spend more time with his children and that he wanted to become more involved in church activities. While work-related problems needed to become a focal part of therapy, the Role Checklist nevertheless provided a very practical starting point for the therapeutic process.

Summary

This chapter described the development, preliminary psychometric examination, clinical use, and early research with the Role Checklist. The checklist was developed in response to a need for an efficient assessment of roles in occupational therapy patients. The written inventory elicits the respondent's perceived role incumbency along a temporal continuum in 10 roles as well as the degree to which each role is valued. Data from the instrument provide information about role incumbency, valuation of roles, role balance, and future orientation.

A preliminary study of the test-retest reliability of the Role Checklist indicated that the instrument is satisfactorily stable with a group of normal adults. Content validity of the instrument was based on a review of social psychology and occupational therapy literature. Although concurrent validity with other measures of time organization and role performance has not yet been examined, there is some preliminary evidence that the instrument can discriminate between subjects with adaptive behavior and those with maladaptive behavior. Further, empirical evidence of a relationship between occupational role involvement and life satisfaction lends support to a basic philosophical assumption of occupational behavior.

Empirical assessment of reliability with patient populations needs to be examined. In addition, the reliability of the present version of the religious participant role should be evaluated. Studies of concurrent validity, some of which are presently underway, could be planned using such instruments as the Occupational History and the Occupational Questionnaire to provide data on past and present role incumbency. Long-term studies may be useful to verify if the future perceived incumbency of respondents does indeed predict future role performance or the preparation to enter roles.

In clinical use, the instrument is easy to administer and to interpret. The checklist format presents clients with a visual and concrete image of problems or conflicts in role performance and discrepancies between role incumbency and valued roles. It is hoped that normative data soon will be available to provide a basis of comparison for further interpretation of the instrument.

References

1. Oakley F (1982). The Model of Human Occupation in Psychiatry. Unpublished master's project, Medical College of Virginia, Virginia Commonwealth University, Richmond, Virginia.
2. Kielhofner G and Burke J (1980). A model of human occupation, Part 1. Conceptual framework and content. Am J Occup Ther 34, 572-581.
3. Kielhofner G and Burke J (1985). Components and determinants of occupation, in Kielhofner G (ed): A Model of Human Occupation: Theory and Application. Baltimore: Williams and Wilkins.
4. Reed KL (1984). Models of Practice in Occupational Therapy. Baltimore: Williams and Wilkins.
5. Goffman E (1959). The Presentation of Self in Everyday Life. Garden City, New York: Doubleday Anchor Books.
6. Heard C (1977). Occupational role acquisition: A perspective on the chronically disabled. Am J Occup Ther 31, 243-247.
7. Barris R, Kielhofner G, and Watts J (1983). Psychosocial Occupational Therapy: Practice in a Pluralistic Arena. Laurel, Maryland: Ramsco.
8. Rogers JC (1983). The study of human occupation, in Kielhofner G (ed): Health Through Occupation: Theory and Practice in Occupational Therapy. Philadelphia: F.A. Davis.
9. Reilly M (1969). The educational process. Am J Occup Ther 23, 299-307.
10. Black M (1976). The occupational career. Am J Occup Ther 30, 225-228.
11. Moorhead L (1969). The occupational history. Am J Occup Ther 23, 329-334.
12. Florey L and Michelman S (1982). Occupational role history: A screening tool for psychiatric occupational therapy. Am J Occup Ther 36, 301-308.

13. Kielhofner G, Harlan B, Bauer D, and Maurer P (1986). The reliability of a historical interview with physically disabled respondents. Am J Occup Ther 40, 551-556.
14. Black M (1976). Adolescent role assessment. Am J Occup Ther 30, 73-79.
15. Dunning H (1972). Environmental occupational therapy. Am J Occup Ther 26, 292-298.
16. Fleiss J (1981). Statistical Methods for Rates and Proportions (2nd ed). New York: John Wiley and Sons.
17. Landis J and Koch G (1977). The measurement of observer agreement for categorical data. Biometrics 33, 159-174.
18. Smyntek L, Barris R, and Kielhofner G (1985). The model of human occupation applied to psychosocially functional and dysfunctional adolescents. Occupational Therapy and Mental Health 5, 21-40.
19. Barris R, Kielhofner G, Burch Martin RM, Gelinas I, Klement M, Schultz B. Occupational function and dysfunction in three groups of adolescents. Occupational Therapy Journal of Research. 6, 301-307.
20. Duellman M, Barris R, Kielhofner G (1986). Organized activity and the adaptive status of nursing home residents. Am J Occup Ther 40, 618-622.
21. Elliot MS (1984). Occupational Role Performance and Life Satisfaction in the Elderly. Unpublished master's thesis, Medical College of Virginia, Virginia Commonwealth University, Richmond, Virginia.
22. Versluys H (1980). The remediation of role disorders through focused group work. Am J Occup Ther 34, 609-614.
23. Gray M (1972). Effects of hospitalization on work-play behavior. Am J Occup Ther 26, 180-185.
24. Lamb H (1982). Young adult chronic patients: The new drifters. Hospital and Community Psychiatry 33 465-468.
25. Matsutsuyu J (1969). The interest checklist. Am J Occup Ther 23, 323-328.
26. Kielhofer G and Neville A (1983). Revised version of the interest checklist. Unpublished manuscript, available from authors.
27. Riopel N (1982). An examination of the occupational behavior and life satisfaction of the elderly. Unpublished master's project, Medical College of Virginia, Virginia Commonwealth University, Richmond, Virginia.

CHAPTER 6

THE NPI INTEREST CHECK LIST

Joan C. Rogers, PhD, OTR

Activity selection in occupational therapy often begins with the question: What are you interested in? or What would you like to do? To interest is "to attract and hold attention".[1] In treatment, occupational therapists use interests to engage a patient's attention. The therapeutic objective is to divert a patient's attention from unhealthy thoughts, such as fascination with psychiatric symptomatology, to healthy preoccupations, such as knitting a sweater. Interests are used to manage time productively and to build skill.

Despite the centrality of interests to practice, the concept of interests and its application to patient treatment was not systematically developed in the occupational therapy literature until the late 1960s. In 1968, Matsutsuyu formulated a conceptual perspective of interests and devised the Neuropsychiatric Institute (NPI) Interest Check List to assess the activity preferences of patients.

The purpose of this chapter is to: explain the conceptual basis of interest and interest assessment; describe the most widely used clinical instrument for assessing interest, the NPI Interest Check List; indicate the scientific properties of this instrument; and indentify and analyze critical issues surrounding interest assessment.

The Concept of Interest

Matsutsuyu[2] viewed interest as a facet of personality involved with feeling. A salient feature of individuality is the interests one has. There is a uniqueness about each individual and a part of this uniqueness is attributed to interests. John's attraction to golf may be equal to Paul's dislike for the same activity. Thus, interests may be viewed as differentiating human characteristics.

Interests relate to the affective response to activities. This affect may be positive or negative and the mature personality is able to identify both likes and dislikes. There is an awareness or "self-knowledge" of activities that attract and those that repel. The capability to state preferences is gauged by one's ability to discern the degree to which various activities are liked or disliked.

Interests have their origins in early childhood experiences. Some may emerge from biological predispositions or propensities. For example, Jack may delight in the tactile sensation afforded by sand or mud play. The family unit serves as the primary socializing agent of interests. As the child directs attention to an activity, this attention may be approved or redirected. As attention is channelled, interests are differentiated and patterns developed. Since family members are apt to direct a child's attention to activities that they find pleasurable, interest patterns within families are likely to be more similar than those between other social units.

Among the earliest differentiation of interests to take place is the degree to which attention is focused on persons or objects. This sets into motion a differential tendency to find satisfaction in human or object relations. The socialization process includes being sensitized to societal impressions of appropriate "feminine and masculine" interests.

As one matures, gains experience or is exposed to different opportunities, interest preferences may change. Some interests are developmentally based and await the maturation and learning associated with the development of physical, cognitive and social skills. Thus, interest in strategy games is preceded by preferences for activities involving physical prowess, and cooperative play is preceded by parallel play.

Peer and cultural factors also may have a strong impact on interest development, as is currently evidenced in the popularization of physical fitness, computer literacy, and "Cabbage Patch" dolls. Although interest formation continues throughout life, the exploratory process is heightened during adolescence and interests are relatively more stable throughout adulthood.

Interests have both a subjective and objective component. When a person says, "I am interested in bowling," he is stating a subjective impression. This is called an expressed interest. This same person may go on to comment, "but I have never bowled." The person is thus indicating that interest is based only on thoughts or ideas about the activity, since he lacks the concrete experience of "doing" the activity. Interests that are expressed in activity are called objectified interests. It is important to recognize that, while interests have the potential for leading one to participate in an activity, the mere expression of interest does not mean that participation has occurred. "Trying out" an expressed interest through actual participation may convert an expressed interest to an aversion. Interests that have not been "tried out" have a quality of vagueness, since there has been no opportunity to test one's aptitude for the action involved in the interest. Through experience, one's skills for engaging in the action are identified and refined, and one's response to the activity in terms of pleasure is clarified. This, in turn, leads to increased interest or disinterest and subsequent choices generate from the accumulation of experience.

Interests have the capability of sustaining action as well as evoking it. If an activity is of interest, one will participate in it frequently and persist in doing it, despite discomfort or frustration. If interest wanes, participation is decreased. Persistence is associated with the feelings of pleasantness, enjoyment, satisfaction, accomplishment or purposefulness that are derived from activity engagement. These positive feelings may stem from the action involved in the activity, as is the case when skill is being developed, or from the quality of the end product or result of the action. Presumably, the degree of persistence is related to the strength of positive effect.

It is the capacity of interests to both obtain and sustain attention that allows learning to proceed. As long as interest is maintained, action continues and skill development takes place. Competence emerges as individuals test their abilities, learn about their talents and weaknesses, and develop an image of themselves as successful. The adaptive skills that emerge through the pursuit of interests support the tasks and responsibilities inherent to adult work and family roles. Thus, the occupational therapist's interest in interests is not just to occupy time productively, but to elicit and enhance normal human development processes.

Matsutsuyu[2] summarized the view of interests in six statements:
1. Interests are family influenced
2. Interests evoke affective response
3. Interests are choice states
4. Interests can be manifested in effective action
5. Interests can sustain action
6. Interests reflect self-perception

Further refinement of interest concepts was undertaken by Kielhofner and associates in the specification of the model of human occupation.[3] In the model, interests are regarded as subcomponents of the volition subsystem, or that aspect of humans that has responsibility for determining conscious choice. Interests were defined as "personal dispositions to find pleasure in certain objects, events, or people"[3] (p. 577).

Interests are most apparent in occupational choices in which the individual has the most freedom to choose. Leisure occupations are based almost solely on interest, while work occupations reflect more of a compromise between values, interests, abilities and job opportunities.

The orientation to pleasure is reflected in three dimensions of interest: discrimination, pattern and potency.[3] Discrimination refers to the ability to state a preference for certain occupations. The discrimination of interests is expressed when activities are ranked or prioritized. One might stipulate, for example, "I like to go shopping more than going to the movies." Discrimination includes the ability to discern likes and dislikes, as well as the degree or magnitude of liking or disliking. The ability to detect the reason why an activity is pleasurable is also a facet of discrimination. For instance, the enjoyment of shopping may come from having something new to wear, the challenge of getting the most for your money or the opportunity to meet people. It is hypothesized that the quality of the activity that is associated with pleasure may provide a more salient clue to activity choice than the activity itself.

The second dimension of interests, pattern, refers to the overall configuration of interests. An individual may have a preference for solitary activities such as reading or collecting stamps. To satisfy the need to be with others, however, interest may be developed in a social activity, such as a stamp club or volleyball. While the discrimination of interests may emerge from underlying dispositions for obtaining pleasure, it is likely that the overall pattern of interests is determined by the need for variety and balance in activity choices.

Potency takes into account the connection between expressed interest and participation. This dimension examines the degree to which interests are rooted in experience. Past, present and planned participation patterns are of interest. The activity history furnishes valuable information about discarded interests that can be potentially renewed and about the individual's abilities. When combined with present interests and participation patterns, historical data enable one to trace change and stability in occupational choice. The future is tapped in planned or projected interests, which give a perspective of the skills the individual would like to acquire.

Patients seen in occupational therapy are often characterized by dysfunctions in interest discrimination, pattern and potency. Depressed patients, for example, frequently complain that nothing interests them, that they do nothing for "fun," that no activity gives them pleasure and that they do not care or are unable to do anything. Such patients either lack interests or are unable to discriminate activity preferences. When interests are lacking or ambiguous and ill-defined, activity selection and participation lacks commitment. It becomes difficult to concentrate on an occupation that one cares little about or is "disinterested" in. The potential for experiencing pleasure is constrained and the effect associated with the activity is bland.

For some patients, interest dysfunction emerges in an imbalanced pattern of interests rather than discrimination. The "workaholic" who concentrates all energies around work functions, represents one kind of pattern disorder. The polar opposite, the "leisure-holic," appears to be unable to accept worker responsibilities and focuses energy on recreational pursuits. Interest dysfunction is also exhibited by individuals who engage only in solitary and sedentary activities and neglect social and active needs.

The link between interest and activity is often abruptly severed with traumatic conditions such as spinal cord injury and stroke. As a result of trauma, the patient loses the physical capacity to continue to carry out the activity. Interest can no longer lead to action, or at least not to the same type of action. With progressively degenerating conditions, the link between interest and action is lost more slowly. These examples illustrate the concept of expressed interests that lack potency of present experience.

The NPI Interest Check List

Historical Development

The NPI Interest Check List was developed for use with adult psychiatric patients at the Neuropsychiatric Institute of the University of California at Los Angeles. Although it was originally introduced to aid in program planning decisions, its value for individual therapeutic purposes became readily apparent. The instrument was subsequently revised by Matsutsuyu[4] based on findings from clinical usage and interest assessment tool guidelines discussed by Roe and Seligmann[5] and Tyler and Sundberg.[6] The stated purpose of the NPI Interest Check List is to classify and describe the interest state of psychiatric patients.[2] Classification takes into consideration the intensity and types of interests. Description encompasses the individual's ability to express preferences and to discriminate type and intensity.

Description of the Instrument

The NPI Interest Check List has four parts. The first part records identifying information such as the patient's name, the psychiatric unit and the date that the form was completed. Part two is the Check List itself and consists of 80 activity items. The activity choices are presented in writing as opposed to pictures or diagrams. A staccato writing style, such as "gardening" and "poker" is used. This is in contrast to a humanistic writing style, such as "spending time in the garden" or "playing a challenging game of poker." The activity choices are arranged randomly. Again, this format might be contrasted to an alphabetical or categorical (i.e., games, sports, crafts) ordering scheme.

The type of information sought by the Check List is the respondent's present intensity or strength of interest. The directions ask the respondent to "check each item below according to your interest." Responses are arranged in columns labelled "casual, strong, and no," in that order.

For the purposes of interpretation, the 80 items are logically sorted into five categories—Activities of Daily Living (12 items), Manual Skills (12 items), Cultural and Education (12 items), Physical Sports (12 items), and Social Recreational (32 items). The number of casual, strong, and no preferences in each category is ascertained. Weinstein[7] provided the following conceptual definitions of these categories:

Activities of Daily Living refers to the basic domestic arts.

Manual Skills refers to activities that incorporate the use of the hands in making a finished product.

Cultural/Educational refers to activities relating to the training, development and refinement of the mind and mental faculties through systematic study.

Physical Sports refers to activities that incorporate games or play requiring physical strength, agility or stamina.

Social Recreation refers to activities that necessitate participation with other people or are pursued for pleasurable exercise or occupation.

The five categories enable patients' interests to be interpreted in terms of the ability to make discriminative choices and of an interest profile. For example, a patient may exhibit strong interests in one or two categories, or may exhibit no strong interests and have casual interests scattered over all five categories.

Part three of the NPI Interest Check List consists of the open-ended statement, "Please list other special interests." It is intended to account for interests not included on the list. In part four, respondents are asked to describe their interests, hobbies, and pasttimes from grammar school days to the present.

The NPI Interest Check List has been modified in several ways for use in research studies.[8,9] In terms of content, these modifications have reduced the number of activity choices, for example, from 80 items to 68, and refined the phrasing of some items, for instance, changing the term "languages" to "foreign languages." The response format has been expanded to consider interests over the past year, over the past 10 years, in the future, and current participation. Intensity of interest at each time interval was quantified as strong, some, and no.

Administration

The instrument is self-administered. However, if the respondent has any questions about completing the form, clarification may be given. No time limitation is imposed.

Scoring

Scoring is done by hand. Scoring overlays, which highlight the items in each of the five categories, may be constructed to ease scoring. A numerical count of the number of casual, strong, and no interests in each of the categories is obtained. Table 6-1 lists the activity items in each category and numbers each item according to the order in which it is presented on the check list (Appendix C).

Interpretation of Findings

The respondent's choice state is indicated by the intensity of interest (casual, strong, no) expressed for the various activity items. Using these response options, the patient's affective quality of attraction or aversion to an activity item can be described.

The respondent's type of interest is classified according to the five categories. The number of items checked in each category and the intensity of those interests gives an indication of the direction of the patient's interests.

Data from the check list, special interests, and interest history are combined. They are used to prepare a descriptive analysis of the patient's interest state.

The NPI Interest Check List is to be used in concert with other evaluation instruments, rather than as an isolated tool. It is one of several instruments designed by Mary Reilly and associates to aid clinicians in operationalizing occupational behavior concepts. Occupational behavior is defined as the unique balance of work, rest, and play activities created by each individual to accommodate and integrate various life functions and roles. Occupational therapy practice emerging from the occupational behavior frame of reference involves the creation of a laboratory for the exercise of life skills. Interest is one of the core concepts of occupational behavior. Occupational therapy intervention stimulates the development of self-knowledge, individuality, and task skills through interests, while concomitantly allowing for age, sex, and occupational factors and fostering a balance of work, leisure, and rest.

Thus, clinically, the yield from the NPI Interest Check List is to be interpreted in the light of its conceptual basis and in conjunction with the data from other instruments designed to evaluate occupa-

Table 6-1
NPI Interest Checklist Categories,
Activity Items, and Order of Presentation

Manual (12 items)

Activity	Order
sewing	2
car repair	8
needlework	11
manual arts	28
model building	36
woodworking	43
jewelry making	47
leatherwork	56
painting	59
mosaics	66
politics	67

Physical Sports (12 items)

Activity	Order
golf	12
football	13
swimming	20
shuffleboard	31
baseball	37
exercise	41
volleyball	42
billiards	44
tennis	48
basketball	50
ping pong	55

Activities of Daily Living (12 items)

Activity	Order
mending	23
ironing	32
floor mopping	35
home repairs	40
driving	45
dusting	46
cooking	49
shopping	57
laundry	64
decorating	69
clothes	75
hairstyling	77

Table 6-1 *(continued)*
NPI Interest Checklist Categories,
Activity Items, and Order of Presentation

Cultural/Education (12 items)

languages	4
writing	9
lectures	19
reading	26
social studies	33
classical music	34
history	51
science	53
concerts	61
politics	67
math	70
religion	78

Social Recreation (32 items)

gardening	1
poker	3
social clubs	5
radio	6
bridge	7
dancing	1
popular music	14
puzzles	15
holidays	16
solitaire	17
movies	18
visiting	22
chess	24
barbecues	25
traveling	27
parties	29
dramatics	30
checkers	38
singing	39
guitar	52
collecting	54
photography	58
television	60
camping	63
dating	65
Scrabble	68
service groups	71
piano	72
scouting	73
plays	64
drums	79
conversation	80

tional behavior variables, such as the Occupational History[10] and the Decision Making Inventory.[11]

Validation of the expressed interests of patients occurs through a convergence of information obtained through subsequent interviews and the observation of manifest behavior during the course of hospitalization. The NPI Interest Check List also serves as a data base for further inquiry about the patient's interests. For example, knowing the patient's interests, the therapist may explore such questions as: When was the last time you did this activity? How often do you participate in this activity? Is this as frequently as you would like to participate? Did you participate in this activity alone or with others? How would you rate your skill in performing this activity? What is it about this activity that gives you pleasure? Do you do this activity in your home or outside your home? Is there anything that prevents you from participating in this activity? When and how did you learn to do this activity? Such questions clarify and elaborate on the patient's interest state and enable the therapist to formulate a more adequate impression of the patient's interest state.

Research

Reliability

Weinstein[7] obtained a reliability coefficient of 0.92 for the NPI Interest Check List as a whole, using the test-retest methodology. There was a three-week interval between test administrations. The reliability coefficients obtained for each of the interest categories were: 0.84 for Activities of Daily Living; 0.91 for Cultural and Educational; 0.86 for Manual Skills; 0.87 for Social Recreation; and 0.92 for Physical Sports. Thus, the reliability of the overall instrument and of the categories is adequate for making decisions about groups of patients. When making individual, clinical decisions regarding patients, a reliability coefficient of at least 0.90 is recommended. The instrument as a whole meets this criterion.

The subjects used for the reliability study were 48 11th and 12th grade summer school students, residing in Southern California. A modified version of the NPI Interest Check List was used. The response format was expanded from three to six response options. The response options were: like very much, indifferent, dislike, dislike very much, and do not understand what the activity is. These changes were introduced because clinical use of the instrument suggested that the meaning of the term "casual" was ambiguous and difficult to explain. Also, the "strong" and "casual" responses seemed to offer two positive response options, while the "no" was the only negative option. The test taker was thus presented with an unequal number of negative and positive choices. This format could hamper the discrimination of liking and disliking an activity. The five-point rating scale, with equal numbers of like and dislike options and a neutral point, assists the respondent in selecting an answer that is closest to his true feeling about the activity. The response option "do not understand what the activity is" was included because one of the objectives of the study was to ascertain if the activities comprising the check list were appropriate for adolescents.

Content Validity

The content of the NPI Interest Check List was determined on an a priori and clinical basis by experienced occupational therapists. The three criteria used to select activities were: 1) that the activities be commonly understood; 2) that each activity fit into one of the following categories—Manual Skills, Physical Sports, Social Recreation, Activities of Daily Living, or Cultural/Educational; and 3) that participating in the activity be feasible within the hospital program.

The clinical nature of the instrument is evident in the third criterion, namely that participation in the activity be feasible within the hospital program. The NPI Interest Check List was designed to facilitate clinical programming. The intent of the instrument was not to appraise interests in general, but rather to delineate those interests that could be used in treatment. If participation in an activity was not possible within the hospital milieu, which included resources in occupational therapy, therapeutic recreation, and the surrounding hospital and university environment, the activity was not included in the check list.

In appraising the content validity of the instrument for use with normal adolescents, Weinstein[7] found that water skiing, snow skiing, horseback riding, and skateboard riding were interests that were frequently added in response to the inquiry about special interests. These activities might be added to the Physical Sports Category, when the NPI Interest Check List is used with adolescents.

Activity items that were confusing to the subjects were: bridge, mosaics, shuffleboard, and billiards by girls, and mending and jewelry making by boys. Confusion could be reduced by clarifying the nature of these activities in the initial instructions. Subsequent study of the instrument with adolescents may suggest deletion from the list.

Construct Validity

Although no other studies have been conducted specifically to establish construct validity, research use of modified versions of the NPI Interest Check List with various populations is beginning to yield evidence of its discriminative capabilities. The available studies furnish suggestions for designing studies to test explicit hypotheses about group differences.

Barris and colleagues[12] found that the number of strong interests in the past 10 years was one of the variables that differentiated normal (N = 10), emotionally disturbed (N = 10), and medically ill (N = 10) adolescents. Emotionally disturbed and medically ill adolescents identified more strong past interests than did the normal adolescents. No differences were seen regarding strong interests one year ago, present enacted interests, or future interests. However, in another study involving adolescents[13] no meaningful differences were detected between psychosocially functional and dysfunctional (N = 37) adolescents in terms of number of interests over the past 10 years, over the past year, or anticipated. Although the dysfunctional subjects had enacted fewer present interests, this finding could be attributed to hospitalization as readily as the psychiatric disorder.

Scaffa[9] investigated interests in alcoholic (N = 25) and non-alcoholic (N = 25) groups. No significant differences were noted between groups in the number of strong interests or in the categories of activities of daily living, manual skills, physical sports, or social recreation. The alcoholic subjects expressed less interest in cultural and educational activities than the non-alcoholic subjects. The subjects were also participating in a narrower range of activities. Overall, while the interests patterns of the alcoholic and non-alcoholic groups were highly similar, the level of participation of the alcoholic subjects was markedly lower than the non-alcoholic subjects.

NPI Interest Check List data also entered into the analysis performed by Oakley, Keilhofner, and Barris[14] to appraise the organization of the volition subsystem and the human system as a totality. The subjects (N = 30) had various psychiatric diagnoses. Interest patterns were so variable that group trends were not discernible.

Kavanaugh, Barris, and Kielhofner[15] selected 40 activities from the NPI Interest Check List to use with mentally retarded adults (N = 23). As photographs of each activity were presented, the subjects responded in terms of interest or non-interest. A significant association emerged between interests and degree of competent participation in sheltered workshop, leisure, and home settings.

Owens[16] explored the use of the NPI Interest Check List with subjects with a medical rather than a psychiatric diagnosis. The interests of spinal cord injured persons (N = 30) were studied in relation to a number of variables. Daily productivity of the subjects was not correlated with the number of interests rated "like" or "like very much." A significant correlation with productivity was found when interests were associated with future goals. In interpreting these findings, the authors suggested that the mere quantification of interests is probably not an acceptable methodology, since numbers of interests may not be indicative of healthy functioning. The fact that interests assume significance in the context of goals implies that it is the "overall meaningfulness of the activities" that comprise one's lifestyle that is important.

Limitations in Interest Assessment

A critical issue surrounding the use of any instrument is the validity and reliability of the data generated. Validity involves the extent to which an instrument measures what it purports to measure. An instrument is not inherently valid. It may be valid for some uses and not for others.

When a check list is devised, some choices must be made regarding the activities to include and exclude. It is not feasible to present the respondent with an "endless" list of activities. The number of activities presented must be limited in some way. When constructing an activity list, a balance is sought in terms of formulating a list that is not so long that it becomes unmanageable, and one that is not so short that it furnishes little descriptive information. In accordance with its clinical utility, the NPI Interest Check List was constructed to include activities that were available at the Institute or in the surrounding community. Thus, in applying this instrument to other settings, serious consideration must be given to the content validity of the test. The activity items may not be applicable to other settings or populations. The establishment of content validity is essentially a judgmental process. The potential test user reviews the activity list and makes an appraisal of its utility in the proposed setting.

Concerns about data reliability focus on the stability of measurement. If therapeutic activities are to be selected on the basis of interest assessment, therapists need assurance that the patient's measured interests represent real interests and are not a reflection of measurement error. If a patient's interest profile indicated a strong positive feeling for physical sports on Monday morning and an equally strong negative feeling for the same activities on Monday afternoon, the interest inventory would be of little value as a starting point for treatment planning. This inventory would be regarded as unreliable. A stable measure of interests is needed to take advantage of the motivational potential of interests.

The stability of subjects' responses over time to the NPI Interest Check List was established only in regard to a small sample of normal adolescents. There is a critical need to establish reliability in regard to patient populations. Interest assessment generally is undertaken in conjunction with the initial occupational therapy assessment, and one can legitimately question the degree to which a patient who is acutely psychotic or has only recently been paralyzed can give reliable information. One approach to reliability appraisal would be to ascertain the agreement between the patient's expressed interests and interests as described by knowledgeable informants such as family members. Another approach would involve comparing interest data collected initially, during the acute phase of illness, or early stage of rehabilitation, with that collected when behavior has become more stabilized.

Reliance on the check list format (part two), rather than an unstructured, open-ended format, such as that used in parts three and four, improves reliability. The check list requires the respondent to recognize interests, while the open-ended question necessitates recall. Anyone who has had experience with sentence completion (i.e., fill-in-the-blank) and multiple-choice type questions knows that recognition is easier than recall. Providing a memory aid, such as a check list, may be particularly valuable for cognitively impaired individuals or those under severe stress.

Inclusion of the open-ended question encourages respondents to consider interests not on the list. Thus, it picks up activity preferences that are less common or normative. Having been exposed to the check list activity items before the open-ended question, respondents are sensitized to the kind of information wanted. Thus, it is often easier to think about activity preferences after having gone through the check list than it was beforehand. Systematic review of the number and pattern of items volunteered by various groups in response to the open-ended question provides a mechanism for establishing and updating content validity.

Adaptations of the NPI Interest Check List were introduced to measure various aspects of the activity items. In its original version, the instrument measured the intensity of interest, or how much interest the individual had in each activity item. The original response format of "strong, casual, no" has been varied to include "strong, some, no" and "like very much, like, indifferent, dislike, and dislike very much." Although a gradation of response options increases the sensitivity of measurement, it also increases the complexity of the task. The most rudimentary measurement is the simple occurrence of a behavior. It is easier to say "yes, I like to swim" or "no, I do not like to swim," than it is to judge whether you "like to swim" or "like very much to swim." Use of the pictorial format in conjunction with the "yes or no" response options, was directed toward simplifying the assessment process for the mentally retarded individuals studied by Kavanagh, Barris, and Kielhofner.[15]

Another approach to ascertaining intensity of interest is to prioritize one's preferences. This approach could be combined with check list use. For example, after respondents have delineated strong interests, they might rank order them from most to least preferred. This procedure would yield additional information on activity preferences.

To gauge changes over time in activity choices and in level of interest in regard to particular activities, a retrospective measurement technique has been used. Respondents are asked to think back one year, ten years, or to pre-injury status, and rate the items as they would have at that time. This procedure is used to gain a longitudinal view of the respondent's interests. In effect, this procedure structures part four of the original instrument in which respondents were asked to describe interests from elementary school to the present. Retrospective measurement should be used cautiously. The cognitive capacity of respondents to retrospect may be limited. For example, when 15-year-old adolescents are asked to go back in time 10 years, they are challenged to recall interests at 5 years of age. In addition to questioning their ability to recall this information, one must also consider the adequacy of the NPI Interest Check List, an inventory of adult interests, for delineating the interests of 5 year olds.

Retrospective measurement also raises multiple questions concerning respondent bias. For example, in reflecting on pre-injury status, it is conceivable that an individual might perceive more interest or involvement than he actually had or did. This bias would serve to make the discrepancy between pre-injury and post-injury status wider than it actually was. Thus, while retrospective measurement may be an adequate measure of the respondent's perceptions of change and stability, it may be a poor indicator of actual behavioral change.

Although participation is a commonly used index of interest, its use has been highly criticized. Participation in activities, or the ability to pursue one's interests, may be constrained by multiple things. McGuire,[17] for example, found considerable discrepancy between the actual and desired participation of older adults. While they were involved in solitary and sedentary activities, they preferred to be involved in social and more active activities. The subjects were unable to pursue interests because of poor health; a lack of transportation, money, skill, companionship or facilities; a sense that they were too old to learn new activities; and a fear of disapproval from family and friends. Fundamental to interest assessment is a keen appreciation of the distinction between expressed and objectified interests or, in other words, of the discrimination and potency dimensions of interest.

Interpretation of the NPI Interest Check List is aided by grouping the activity items according to common characteristics. Matsutsuyu[2] selected activities of daily living, manual skills, cultural and education, physical sports, and social recreation as the major organizational concepts. While Rogers, Weinstein, and Figone[18] detected some problems with this scheme based on empirical testing, research requires replication before instrument revision is warranted. Furthermore, the underlying empirical structure does not destroy the logical basis for item groupings. Other common coding schemes for interpreting discrete items are: an emphasis on physical as opposed to mental activity, sometimes interpreted as active and passive interests; interests carried out indoors as opposed to those out-of-doors; and interests that are pursued alone as opposed to those done with others.

A final consideration in regard to interest assessment is the respondent's overall orientation to self-maintenance, work, and leisure occupations. The major yield from the NPI Interest Check List is attitudes toward specific occupations. From a more general perspective, it is important to know the relative value that the respondent places on these three occupational categories. It is for interpretive purposes that interest data are placed in the context of other evaluative data and ultimately of the occupational behavior frame of reference.

Further Research

The test author, Matsutsuyu,[2] suggested that the relationship between interest patterns, as evaluated by the NPI Interest Check List, and personality structure, as measured by the Minnesota Multiphasic Personality Inventory, be studied. If personality and interests were found to be related, the study would provide one explanation of the meaning of interest patterns. Since the Minnesota Multiphasic Personality Inventory has been correlated with other interest instruments, such as the Strong Vocational Interest Blank and the Kuder Preference Record, such an investigation would also explore the validity of the NPI Interest Check List.

Adoption of the NPI Interest Check List for clinical or research use requires evidence of its appropriateness for use with the proposed population. As evidence of the instrument's capacity to differentiate clinical and normal groups, and various diagnostic categories accumulate, hypothesis testing studies can be conducted. These investigations will contribute to construct validity. A neglected area of interest research is the meaning of activity choices. Since meaning is inherent to the therapeutic selection of occupation, this aspect of interests reflects a research priority.

Summary

An interest is a choice state reflecting a positive attitude toward an activity. Pleasure may be derived from the action involved in the activity or the end product emerging from the action. The family serves as a primary socializing agent for interests. The child's interests are channelled by parents, siblings, and other family members who approve of some activities and disapprove of or fail to support others. One major orientation that is reinforced within the family is a preference for activities focused on humans in contrast to objects. Some interests are developmentally based and await the maturation of physical, mental, and social capabilities. The formation of interests is also strongly influenced by peer pressure and cultural trends. Adolescence is a time of extensive leisure exploration. Throughout adulthood, interests and participation patterns are more stable.

In occupational therapy, interests are used to attract and hold attention so that time may be used effectively to learn skills. Skill learning may be directed toward the leisure activity itself, as in a case when the treatment objective involves learning to play bridge well enough to join a bridge club so that social needs may be satisfied. Or, skill learning may be directed toward the motor, cognitive, or social components of the activity, as is the case when the treatment objective involves relearning fine motor skills by manipulating playing cards. Thus, interests are used to foster the emergence of competence.

The effective use of interests in treatment depends on an adequate assessment of interests. The interest assessment covers the discrimination, pattern, and potency of interests, as well as changes in these dimensions over time and as a consequence of impairment. Interest discrimination is the ability to state activity preferences. The extent to which expressed interests are participated in is referred to as potency of interests. The pattern of interests involves the configuration of expressed and objectified interests. Dysfunction may be evidenced in one or all three interest dimensions.

The NPI Interest Check List, a four-part, self-administered instrument, was devised to facilitate interest assessment. Part one seeks identifying descriptive information about the patient. Part two is the 80-item check list. Each activity is rated by the respondent as casual, strong, or no interest. For the purposes of interpretation, the activity items are classified into one of five categories—Activities of Daily Living, Manual, Cultural and Educational, Physical Sports, and Social Recreation. The check list yields measures of interest discrimination and pattern. Potency is not evaluated by the check list per se, but is generally covered in the follow-up interview, when the instrument is used clinically. Part three appraises special interests not tapped by the check list. In part four, patients record their activity history from grammar school through the present. Data from all four parts of the instrument are combined to furnish a profile of the patient's interest state. The NPI Interest Check List was developed for clinical use with psychiatric patients whose occupational therapy was carried out from an occupational behavior frame of reference.

Little is known about the scientific properties of the NPI Interest Check List. The test-retest reliability coefficient obtained using a modified version of the tool with adolescents was 0.92. Content validity is based on activities available at the Neuropsychiatric Institute of the University of California at Los Angeles when the instrument was developed. Although no studies have been designed to ascertain construct validity, descriptive research points to the strength, range, and types of interests as discriminating variables and suggests that interests be studied in relation to participation and goals.

While the NPI Interest Check List represents the seminal interest tool for occupational therapy, many interest measures and methodologies are available. Instrument selection should be based on the intended use of the information. The check list format has several advantages over an unstructured one. It provides a standardized stimulus for all patients to respond to, and hence improves reliability. The check list also eases the burden on memory, since it requires the recognition of information rather than its recall. This is particularly important when patients are acutely ill or cognitively impaired. In addition, reviewing the activity list sets up expectations in the patient for the type of information desired by the therapist. Hence, when the check list is used in conjunction with open-ended questions, the patient is often better able to respond appropriately.

Since the activity list must be limited in some way, the item content must be critically reviewed for its validity for the use intended. When retrospective measurement is employed, the list of activities must be applicable for the interval covered by retrospection. Adaptations of the NPI Interest Check List illustrate the verbal and pictorial modes of stimulus presentation. Similarly, variations of the response format indicate options for both expressed and objectified interests. To facilitate the interpretations of interest data, interests are categorized according to schemes such as primarily physical or mental activity and activity done alone or with others.

Appraisal of the reliability and validity of the NPI Interest Check List is a high priority for research. Other research suggestions involve exploring the meaning of activity and investigating the relationship between interests and other aspects of occupation and personality.

References

1. Hinsie LE and Campbell RJ (1960). Psychiatric Dictionary. New York: Oxford University Press.
2. Matsutsuyu JS (1968). An Assessment of Interests. Unpublished master's thesis, University of Southern California, Los Angeles.
3. Kielhofner G and Burke JP (1980). A model of human occupation, Part 1: Conceptual framework and content. Am J Occup Ther 34, 572-581.
4. Matsutsuyu JS (1969). The Interest Check List. Am J Occup Ther 23, 368-373.
5. Roe A and Seligman M (1964). The Origins of Interests. Washington D.C.: American Personnel and Guidance Association.
6. Tyler LE and Sundberg ND (1964). Factors Affecting Career Choice of Adolescents. Cooperative Research Project #2455, Eugene University of Oregon.
7. Weinstein J (1979). The Generation of Profiles of Adolescent Interests. Unpublished master's thesis, University of Southern California, Los Angeles.
8. Kielhofner G and Neville A. Revised Version of the Interest Check List. Unpublished manuscript.

9. Scaffa ME (1981). Temporal Adaptation and Alcoholism. Unpublished master's project, Virginia Commonwealth University, Richmond.

10. Moorhead L (1969). The occupational history. Am J Occup Ther 23, 329-334.

11. Westphal M (1967). A Study of Decision Making. Unpublished master's thesis, University of Southern California, Los Angeles.

12. Barris R, Kielhofner G, Burch Martin RM, Gelinas I, Klement M, Schultz B (1986). Occupational function and dysfunction in three groups of Adolescents. Occupational Therapy Journal of Research 6, 301-307.

13. Smyntek L, Barris R, and Kielhofner G (1985). The model of human occupation applied to psychosocially functional and dysfunctional adolescents. Occupational Therapy in Mental Health 5, 21-39.

14. Oakley F, Kielhofner G, and Barris R (1985). An Occupational therapy approach to assessing psychiatric patients' adaptive functioning. Am J Occup Ther 39, 147-154.

15. Kavanagh M, Barris R, and Kielhofner G (1982). Person-Environment Interactions: The Model of Human Occupation Applied to Mentally Retarded Adults. Unpublished master's project, Virginia Commonwealth University, Richmond.

16. Owens JS (1982). A Study of the Occupational Behavior of Physically Disabled Persons: Motivation and Productivity. Unpublished master's thesis, Virginia Commonwealth University, Richmond.

17. McGuire F (1980). The incongruence between actual and desired leisure involvement in advanced adulthood. Activities, Adaptation and Aging 1, 77-89.

18. Rogers JC, Weinstein JM, and Figone, JJ (1978). The interest Check List: An empirical assessment. Am J Occup Ther 32, 628-630.

CHAPTER 7

BARTH TIME CONSTRUCTION

Tina Barth MA, OTR, CRC

The Barth Time Construction (BTC) is a color-coded time chart in which the patient depicts the use of time for a week within 12 categories of activities. Since it has standardized materials and instructions, it is designed to allow independent participation by patients who are consistent with Allen's[1] cognitive Level 4. By providing pre-cut strips of colors and a grid-like chart to complete, it focuses the subject, yet allows free choice as to color, length, and placement of each strip. The resulting chart is a projective functional self-image that is easily quantifiable. The concept of classifying time and time usage patterns has been central to Occupational Therapy since its inception.[2] The BTC allows the therapist to introduce this concept at the initial evaluation stage while gathering a sample of task behavior. The therapist's focus on time usage leads readily into an investigation of roles and underlying habits and skills.[3] This discussion can be the contracting basis for evaluation and treatment with the patient.

Theoretical Base

Reasons for BTC Development

The BTC was developed in an adult psychiatric setting in response to pressing clinical needs to collect more complete information from patients and to engage them actively in treatment. The existing departmental evaluation battery consisted of a self-report form which included an activity configuration,[4,5] a leather project, and an individual interview. Often, the battery was not completed fully either because of patients' resistance to the fine motor task or because patients only marginally completed the activity configuration. The results from the battery were incomplete, difficult to score and interpret, bulky to store, time consuming, and expensive to obtain.

In order to engage the patients more actively in the evaluation, it was first necessary to examine what was being asked, and its effect on the performance. The patients were usually told during the initial session that occupational therapy is based on a communication process between patient and therapist. The role of the evaluation is to collect information about current level of functioning and past history of function.

According to Reilly, participation in an evaluation battery is closer to a substance activity, "work for income," than a choice activity, "recreation and leisure"[6] (p. 64). In this context, the leather task in the original departmental evaluation was asking patients to communicate information and behave in an adult, businesslike manner, but giving them the tools and tasks of a play or leisure setting with which to do it. The message to the patient was dissonant because the contract for interaction and the task presented did not match. Although a fine motor, leisure craft project was not appropriate, the manipulative elements and opportunities for creative problem solving possible with that type of project needed to be maintained. In order to solve this problem, the evaluation needed to employ a task obviously designed as a communication tool, which would be found in a work or adult environment, and which would allow creative problem solving and the manipulation of materials.

Once the questions of communication and appropriateness of the task to the evaluation situation was addressed, it was necessary to examine the complexity of the task itself. Could the patients be expected to complete the task independently? Did it matter to the interpretation or usefulness of the overall evaluation battery if some parts were incomplete? In the case of the activity configuration, it did matter if the information was spotty or unclear. The specific content of the configuration was used as the basis for the next step in the ongoing evaluation process. The situation called for an adaptation of the activity configuration concept into a standardized task, with as simple a procedure as possible to maximize the patient's ability to complete it. The less the therapist intervened in the completion of the task, the more confidence there would be that the product reflected the patient's real functional level and unedited activity preferences.

An activity configuration in a task format with sharp graphics and bright colors would increase patient attention to the task. The task should have a limited array of responses which would be easily quantifiable and contribute directly to the formulation of a treatment plan. The task should include enough choices to allow for creative problem solving in well-constituted patients, but have very clear, simple instructions and presentation of materials to encourage mildly decompensated patients. This time task would represent an adult, work-like communication opportunity, which is completely consistent with the goals of an evaluation session.

Implementation of such a task in the evaluation battery would eliminate several other problems as well. The craft activity would be no longer necessary if enough of the elements it displayed could be incorporated into the time task design. This would mean a decrease in cost for materials and total time to administer the evaluation battery. If the task could be designed to promote participation by cognitively lower functioning patients, the clarity and amount of specific information available from the activity configuration section of the evaluation would increase. When patients are asked clinical questions and are allowed to answer directly with appropriate media, the product requires less therapist interpretation, which often can mean less editing. Representing the patient through product would make an excellent basis for presenting the patient to the rest of the treatment team, as well as demonstrating the nature of occupational therapy. Occupational therapy could be presented as a profession interested in time and a patient's relationship to it, his balance of activities within time, and his ability to perform those activities.

Historic Development

The BTC progressed through three stages in its development. The first stage was characterized by hands-on clinical experimentation. Allen's cognitive disability theories[1] were applied to the Activity Configuration task[4,5] in order to engage chronic schizophrenic patients in reporting more details of their time-usage patterns. The "directions," "color code," and "time chart" parts of the BTC kit were designed and the instructions for administration were written using Allen cognitive level 4 as a guide.[1] All instructions are in declarative style in the present tense. The BTC process only requires working with one dimension at a time—length. Crossing the midline in the vertical field was eliminated; all work to complete the BTC can be done on the midline using a vertical format. Once the format of the forms was set, the color selection and assignment of classes of activities was next.

Bendroth and Southam suggest that patients select colors to reflect mood.[7] In order to test if one color represents an activity more than another, colors for the color code were chosen based on patient consensus. The BTC was used with an inpatient alcoholic population for three months. Patients were presented a time chart and asked to fill it in with pre-cut strips of color to represent how time for a week was spent. After each color was in place, the name of the activity it represented was written on the chart. All the responses were recorded. The color assignments in the color code are those which were most common in that alcoholic population. For example, sleeping was most frequently represented by blue, rather than yellow or orange, thus blue represent sleeping on the color code. Next, the activity categories were examined for content validity.

The second stage in the development of the BTC was characterized by consensus decision making. Once the forms were standardized, the BTC replaced the leather task as part of the occupational therapy departmental evaluation. The COTE Scale[8] was used to score performance. Although the forms were standardized, each therapist who administered the BTC presented the task in a slightly different manner. The written instructions were not specific enough to cover the exceptions and questions that patients and therapists alike were asking about administration and interpretation.

At the same time, the BTC had spread to two more institutions as part of the evaluation batteries. The author formed a supervision workshop with therapists from the three institutions and two therapists in private practice. The Time Construction Workshop met with a group of 15 occupational therapists over a two-year period. These therapists were all concurrently using the BTC as a condition of workshop attendance. Using group consensus, the workshop considered the patients' physical abilities, cognitive levels, language and reading levels. The workshop also explored ways to meet the therapists' own needs to shorten evaluation time, yet improve the quality of information collected. The therapists rewrote the instructions and debated through what became the administration section of the BTC manual. The comments on clinical practice, which appear in the BTC manual section on handling problems with administration, were recorded in this workshop. The result was a tool which is simple to administer to one to six patients at a time, and which nets a task behavior sample and specific individual information at the same time. This information leads directly into treatment planning and leaves the patient with a clear view that the occupational therapist is interested in how one spends time and how satisfied one is with it.

The final stage of BTC development consisted of putting together the pieces and filling the gaps. After the workshop phase, it was clear that the patient information on the time chart would be less valuable if it could not be summarized with a high degree of reliability or communicated efficiently and clearly. The author designed a coding routine for quantifying hours spent in each class of activity by examining over 100 time charts produced by an acute inpatient psychiatric population. Interrater reliability for the scoring procedure was tested.

The author felt that for practical purposes, any summary form should not be more than one page and should hold all the information in its final usable form. Extra time is spent and errors can occur when copying information from one source to another. The BTC Summary Form was designed to include background information on the patient, process notes during BTC administration, a numerical score showing total hours per week spent in each activity, and summary notes or a treatment plan. The summary form can be used for initial data gathering and case presentation. When filed with the time chart, it becomes a data base for research.

The last step involved making or finding all the parts that went into a kit: printed forms in pads, labels for storage boxes, experimenting with laminating directions and color code sheets to make them washable and reusable, getting supplies such as glue bottles and boxes, and finding a supplier for all the colors of paper needed.

Client Population

In adolescent and adult populations, the BTC is used for gathering information on how the patient spends a week of time. The clinical application of this information varies depending on the particular population. In a general psychiatric population of Allen level 4 and above,[1] the BTC can be repeated frequently and used to build time-management skills. It can be used as a time map with which to make abstract concepts concrete.[9] The BTC is entirely consistent with the Activities Configuration[4,5] and can be used to explore issues of autonomy as described in the second step of that procedure.

In an alcohol/substance abuse population, the completed time chart can be used with a patient to confront the denial of the effect of drinking/drugs on the quality of life. Often, when the time necessary for securing and using drinks/drugs is removed, there are large blank areas on the time chart. The BTC can be used as a basis for exploring alternative ways to manage that time. In adolescent populations, time charts can be used in peer group therapy as a basis for identifying mutual areas of concern and problem solving. When the BTC is used with a severely physically disabled adult population, it can be used to assist in beginning working through the denial stage of the grief reaction. It can focus patients on the present physical changes that require shifts in time usage planning as part of a rehabilitation treatment plan.

The BTC is used as a means of operationalizing abnormal or socially unusual patterns of behavior that may warrant further investigation by the treatment staff. Target problem areas for the population are defined. As each time chart is completed, the therapist screens it for problem areas and reports findings to the treatment staff. For example, a possible eating disorder may be indicated by eating as a sole activity more than two hours in a row on more than one occasion during a week. A sleep disorder may be indicated by less than 28 hours or more than 56 hours of sleep per week, or sleeping more than 10 hours in any 24-hour period. An alcohol/drug problem may be indicated by drinking/drugs as a sole activity more than three hours in a row on more than one occasion per week. Currently, the definitions are developed by a treatment team for its particular population. When using the BTC in this way, each treatment team is able to define its own priorities and areas of concern.

The BTC can be used as a means of documenting persons' use of time. It can be used to record changes with individual cases in activity level and balance of activity at several points in occupational therapy treatment. Program effectiveness can be documented by administering a BTC before and after a treatment program and comparing the results. A need for programming can be demonstrated by comparing BTC activity levels and their balance in a population receiving services and a comparable population that is not receiving them. The BTC can be used to gather data for tables of norms of activity balance for any population, e.g., teenagers, homemakers, or senior citizens.

The BTC is useful as a communication tool that graphically demonstrates a patient's level of function, activity balance, and occupational therapy's active relationship to these areas. It is used as a communication tool with the patient by allowing the therapist a means to point out specific examples of strengths and weaknesses in coping patterns and activity balance. When the BTC is combined with the COTE Scale,[8] it is useful in communicating and teaching clinical students observation/evaluation skills for a standardized task. Since time and its usage are central themes in occupational therapy, using an instrument based on these ideas facilitates educating hospital staff to the nature and practice of occupational therapy. The BTC is not only the patient's statement about how he spends time, but also is an example of how he is able to complete a standardized task. When communicating with the treatment team, it can be shown as a clear sample of the patient's level of function. It is also useful when therapists discuss a case successively treated at different sites within a facility, or discuss a patient with a particular diagnosis treated at different facilities.

Review of the Literature

Concerns about man's actual use of time and ability to perform activities that are "helpful and gratifying" was presented as the main tenet of occupational therapy by Meyer in 1922.[2] Since Meyer, occupational therapy has focused on the balance of work, play, ADL, and sleep. Reilly defined this perspective by proposing a theory of human occupation. The author stated that occupational therapists should examine life roles and supporting skills. Treatment should focus on balanced ADL and those skills that pertain to planning and implementing each individual's daily living schedule.[6] Kielhofner developed propositions about the nature of temporal adaptation. The author theorizes that there is a culturally determined temporal frame of reference expressed through acceptable social roles. An individual's use of time is a function of values, interests, and goals. It is maintained through habit structure. Particular pathologies have certain patterns of temporal dysfunction.[9]

In order to understand a patient's temporal dysfunction, it is necessary to know the specifics as to how time is spent. Four evaluations stand out in this respect. The Activity Analysis by Buchenholtz organizes a patient's statements about activity by age level and aspects of the activity. The author used this information to understand the psychodynamic uses of activities in an adolescent psychiatric population.[11] The Activity Configuration method designed by Spahn consists of an initial interview, weekly time chart, self-rating form, and follow-up interview.[4] The specifics of the time chart are recoded into classes of activity. The patient rates his level of autonomy in each class. The Occupational History by Moorhead is used for clinical history taking and is designed to gather information on six different life roles: three main occupational roles, paid employment, housewife, full-time student or student role in general, peer role, and family role.[12] The NPI Interest Check List by Matsutsuyu provides an overview of patients' interest choices within an 80-item list. The items can be grouped into five large categories: manual skills, physical sports, social recreation, ADL, and cultural/educational activities.[13]

Behaviors Assessed

The BTC assesses behavior in three areas. It reliably scores the patient's report on 12 classes of activities engaged in over a one-week period. It combines these findings into percent of time spent in ADL, work, leisure, and sleep. The BTC can be used as the basis of a parallel level task group. By employing the COTE Scale,[8] this group can be used to assess group interaction skills and task skills.

Administration

The Materials

The BTC is available in a kit with supplies to administer it to a maximum of six patients at one group setting. The kit contains pads of forms and laminated reusable instruction sheets; cylindrical glue bottles; 12 packets of colored strips, 1 inch x 12 inches, one color per packet; a clear plastic overlay for scoring; and the BTC manual. Six pairs of right-handed and one pair of left-handed 8-in scissors, eight pencils, and white glue are also required. A clipboard for use by the therapist to hold summary forms during the administration is helpful.

There are four pages of forms. Page 1, "Directions," and page 2, "Color Code," are printed in quarter inch bold type. They are written in simple, declarative, and step-by-step style. They are laminated in heavy non-glare plastic and washable for re-use. Page 3, "Time Chart," is a grid-like form with seven columns of 24 boxes each. Each column of boxes is 1 inch wide. Days of the week are printed across the top in bold print and hourly designations from midnight to 11 PM are printed down the left side. The form is heavy, 90-lb stock that will not curl with large amounts of glue. Page 4, "Summary Form," is a one-page questionnaire designed to record background information, diagnosis; treatment questions; process notes; total hours spent in each category of activity, with a conversion to percent of total time spent in ADL, work, leisure, and sleep; and a summary or treatment plan. The BTC manual contains sections covering the basis of BTC development, directions for set-up, verbal instructions to subjects, verbatim comments from subjects and sample therapist responses, instructions for ending sessions, directions for completing the summary form, a scoring routine for report of time, reliability and validity and a bibliography.

Procedure

The BTC is ideally administered in a group of three to six subjects at one time. If necessary, it can be administered individually. Subjects should be seated around a well-lit large table with a clock visible. Since the BTC requires concentration, it is not recommended to administer it in a day-room setting, unless there is no concurrent activity.

The administration can be broken into three parts. First, prior to the actual group, the therapist completes the top third of a summary form for each subject, which covers demographics, current living conditions, prescribed and non-prescribed drug history, present medications, highest and current level of functioning, and diagnosis. After selecting patients for the group, the therapist prepares the testing table by placing a pair of scissors and a bottle of glue at each place. The packets of colored strips are placed in the middle of the table. The first three pages of forms are collated into packets. If the therapist is using a clipboard to take notes during administration, the summary forms and BTC manual are clipped to it.

The next stage of administration is the group itself. After the subjects arrive in the designated area and are seated at the table, the therapist reads the instructions verbatim from the BTC manual and passes out collated packets of pages 1 to 3. The subjects proceed to complete the time chart at their own pace and have one hour to do so. Subjects are instructed to raise their hands for questions or help, which is given one to one. Any assistance or encouragement given is recorded in the center section of the summary form along with any subject comments. The therapist remains as non-interactive as possible, usually sitting or standing to the side and recording process. Fifteen minutes before the time is up, the therapist reads the instructions from the closure section of the BTC manual and inserts the date and time of the next occupational therapy appointment to go over the time charts.

The last stage of administration occurs after the subjects have left. The therapist cleans and stores the materials according to the BTC checklist. If the BTC is being used as a standardized fine motor task, the therapist completes a COTE Scale[8] for each subject. The therapist scores each time chart by placing the clear plastic overlay on the chart and approximating the hours reported based on the coding frame, "Totaling Hours by Color" in the BTC manual. The bottom third and right side of the summary form are used to record hours reported, the conversion to percent of total time, and any group summary or treatment planning notes. The therapist signs and dates each summary form. The summary form and an attached time chart and COTE Scale[8] can be filed and is readily available without any recoding for consultation with the patient or staff and for research projects.

Problems With Administration

The chief problem areas involve using printed materials, resistance to media other than paper and pencil, and physical limitations which preclude use of scissors, and accurately placing strips of paper. At present, the BTC is available in an English version only. If subjects do not have a reading level sufficient to read the directions and proceed independently, the BTC manual has instructions and examples of how to give verbal aid and demonstration. Some subjects will resist any media other than paper and pencil. The BTC manual has a section with verbatim comments from subjects and sample therapist responses. Often, use of the firm, guiding response to a resistive comment is all that is required to get a subject engaged in the task. In some situations, therapists are more interested in the information the BTC gives than the process of the subject creating it, and find the cutting and pasting cumbersome. Currently, work is underway on the feasibility of developing additional versions of the BTC which are described below.

Utilization of the Assessment

Studies and Statistical Analysis

The scoring criteria detailed in the coding frame were tested for interrater reliability. There is no appreciable difference in scores at the 95% confidence level. Content validity was established using the Activity Analysis,[11] Activity Configuration,[4,5] Occupational History,[12] and NPI Interest Check List[13] to define the behavior domain. For additional details, see the BTC manual.

Interpretation of Results

The BTC can be interpreted from several vantage points: how it was produced, the gestalt of what was produced, and the content of what was produced. When evaluating how the time chart was constructed, the therapist considers performance in task and interpersonal skill areas. These are quantified by the COTE Scale.[8] An area closely related to task skills is the gestalt, one's overall impression of the time chart. This impression can suggest one type of psychopathology more strongly than another. For example, a time chart with some hand-torn pieces of various lengths pasted randomly suggests a subject unable to make the construction. This type of time chart is consistent with a cognitive functional level of 3 rather than 4, which is often found with a psychosis. A time chart that has three or fewer days completed in an hour, with pasting over and tiny pieces all neatly aligned, demonstrates the fussy quality consistent with obsessive-compulsive personality features. A time chart which is completed in 15 to 20 minutes, making no reference to eating, sleeping, or TV, but having at least seven other activity classes depicted, has the frenetic quality consistent with manic personality features. A time chart with strips cut in various lengths, properly aligned, and reference a variety of activities including eating, sleeping, and recreation, would appear in a well population.

The content of the time charts can be investigated given an understanding of the details of each category, as well as the overall balance of classes of activity. As part of a treatment planning session with a patient, the therapist can ask the patient to describe what specific activities are part of a large category, for example, recreation or work. If the subject's explanation is insufficient or unclear, the therapist may pursue the investigation of this area using an instrument designed to elicit more specific responses in a particular area. For example, in the area of worker role, Moorhead's Occupational History[12] is useful.

The therapist can also inquire about a specific activity which is not one of the 12 activity categories listed on the color code, for example, travel, in order to find out how the patient views it. Is it part of the work day? Is it ever/always seen as a separate entity? Is this because it is not integrated as a skill, but is still at the task level? The categorization of activities in the BTC is based on the theory of occupational behavior proposed by Mary Reilly,[6] in which all life activity can be grouped into ADL, work, and choice activities. The balance depicted in a time chart should be investigated for each subject. Proportionately large or small blocks of time assigned to one activity, such as more than 10 hours sleep per day with no physiological abnormalities, are investigated to determine the reason for the apparent imbalance. The reverse is also investigated. Can a subject sustain unstressed function with only five hours sleep per day? How is coping style affected by a report of work for 10 hours per day including weekends? Is it necessary for an individual to practice any home maintenance to achieved adult role status?

Suggestions for Further Research

The forms and procedures of the BTC were developed using Allen's[1] descriptions of function at various cognitive levels. It was assumed that since these guidelines were followed, a BTC time chart can be independently constructed by a person with a functional cognitive level of 4 or higher. Studies to validate the cognitive level requirements of the BTC are needed.

The BTC could be used as a data collection tool for tables of norms showing activity balance for populations by main worker role, psychiatric diagnosis, physical disability, and differences within these groups by age and sex. Time charts could be examined based on descriptive criteria for different gestalts in a blind comparison to DSM III numbers in order to study how task execution may be related to clinical diagnosis.

The BTC could be adapted to reach populations it does not presently serve. Physically disabled patients using ball-bearing feeders after a stroke could benefit from a version of the BTC which used large pens and a three-dimensional chart overlay rather than the colored strips. The same population could use a version employing game pegs and a special board for a time chart. This would give them a reason for picking up and placing in addition to fine motor exercise. There are situations where a functional evaluation is not required and the goal is to maximize the product clarity and minimize the process elements. Research is needed into a BTC version which uses translucent marking pens to color code over written particulars.

References

1. Allen CK (1982). Independence through activity: The practice of occupational therapy. Am J Occup Ther 36, 731-739.
2. Meyer A (1977). The philosophy of occupational therapy. Am J Occup Ther 31, 639-648.
3. Cubie SH, Kaplan K (1982). A case analysis method for the model of human occupation. Am J Occup Ther 36, 645-656.
4. Spahn R (1965). The Patient Gets Busy: Change or Process. Paper presented at March 1965 meeting of the Orthopsychiatric Society, New York.
5. Gillette NP (1971). Occupational therapy and mental health, in Willard HS and Spackman CS (eds). Occupational Therapy (4th ed). Philadelphia: Lippincott.
6. Reilly M (1966). A psychiatric occupational therapy program as a teaching model. Am J Occup Ther 20, 61-67.
7. Bendroth S, Southam M (1973). Objective evaluation of projective material. Am J Occup Ther 27, 78-80.
8. Brayman SJ et al (1976). Comprehensive occupational therapy evaluation scale. Am J Occup Ther 30, 94-100.
9. Neville A (1980). Temporal adaptation: Application with short-term psychiatric patients. Am J Occup Ther 34, 328-331.
10. Kielhofner G (1977). Temporal adaptation: A conceptual framework for occupational therapy. Am J Occup Ther 31, 235-242.
11. Buchenholtz B (1964). Activity analysis: A technique in the study of adolescents. Am J Psychother 18, 594-605.

12. Moorehead L (1969). The occupational history. Am J Occup Ther 23, 329-334.

13. Matsutsuyu JS (1969). The NPI Interest Check List. Am J Occup Ther 23, 323-328.

Bibliography

Allen CK (1985). Occupational Therapy for Psychiatric Diseases: Measurement and Management of Cognitive Disabilities. Boston: Little, Brown and Co.

Barth T (1985). Barth Time Construction. New York: Health Related Consulting Services.

Cynkin S (1979). Occupational Therapy: Toward Health Through Activities. Boston: Little, Brown and Co.

Florey LL and Michelman SM (1982). Occupational role history: A screening tool for psychiatric occupational therapy. Am J Occup Ther 36, 301-313.

Hartocollis P (1976). On the experience of time and its dynamics with special reference to affects. J Am Psychoanal Assoc 24, 363-375.

Hartocollis P (1983). Time and Timelessness: The Varieties of Temporal Experience, a Psychoanalytic Inquiry. New York: International Universities Press.

Loo CM (1974). The self-puzzle: A diagnostic and therapy tool. J Person Assess 38, 236-242.

Reilly M (1974). Play as Exploratory Learning. Beverly Hills, California: Sage Publications.

CHAPTER 8

KOHLMAN EVALUATION OF LIVING SKILLS (KELS)

Linda Kohlman McGourty, MOT, OTR

The Kohlman Evaluation of Living Skills (KELS) is an evaluation designed to assess basic living skills. It is administered by using a combination of interview and task performance techniques. Set-up, administration, and scoring can be completed in 30 to 45 minutes which allows the occupational therapist to develop treatment plans and to assist in discharge planning in a timely manner. The KELS was originally designed to be used for assessing psychiatric inpatients, but it is applicable to a variety of patient populations. Research using small samples has been completed, but the development of the Kohlman Evaluation of Living Skills is an ongoing process. The purpose of this chapter is to describe the historical development of the KELS, the administration and scoring procedures, and results of the research studies. A review of literature is included as well as a discussion of the limitations of this evaluative tool.

Historical Development

The Kohlman Evaluation of Living Skills was first developed in 1978 at Harborview Medical Center in Seattle, Washington. At that time, the author was working on a locked inpatient psychiatric unit. Many of the patients had deficits in living skills and discharge planning was an essential part of the care. The need to systematically assess basic living skills was apparent, but no evaluation tools were available. Typically, each occupational therapist developed his own evaluation method to be used in each individual setting or facility. No consistency between facilities existed and there was questionable reliability within the setting. Most of the evaluations relied entirely on a written format. Therefore, it was difficult to know if a patient had a deficit in living skills. The author identified that some of the psychiatric patients were unable to read and write, but were able to live alone in the community. Others had difficulty reading because of blurred vision due to the side effects of medications. It was important to have an evaluation that identified if a person could read or write, but that would not base the assessment of living skills on that ability. Therefore, the evaluation needed to include other methods besides a solely written format.

Time was another factor. The length of stay for inpatients was starting to decline in 1978 and has continued to decline. Many inpatient psychiatric units operated with high patient volumes and only one occupational therapist. With the shorter length of stay and the high patient case load, the occupational therapist had limited time available to assess patients. It was important to have an evaluation that took a short period of time to administer and score, and yet generated an adequate data base from which to develop treatment and discharge plans.

Another factor that was important to the author in developing the KELS was that the evaluation be easy to administer. With the limited resources of time and energy, the administration process needed to be efficient and not an energy drain for the occupational therapist. Because the setting was a university teaching hospital, students also needed to be able to learn to administer the evaluation and be proficient in a short amount of time.

Communication regarding a patient's status and progress occurs by verbal and written methods on inpatient units. The case load for an occupational therapist can be very high and frequently team conferences occur concurrently. Chart documentation may be the only means of communication available to the occupational therapist. Therefore, the score sheet needed to be easy to understand and short enough so that staff members would read it and use the information.

During the entire development process of the KELS, these factors had been retained to guide the item selection, administration, and scoring process. To summarize, these factors are: 1) high inter-rater reliability; 2) evidence of validity; 3) short set-up, administration, and scoring time; 4) easy administration process; and 5) proficiency in the administration process achieved in a short period of time.

After the development of the Kohlman Evaluation of Living Skills (KELS) for the locked inpatient psychiatric unit at Harborview, other occupational therapists in the Seattle area expressed interest in the KELS and began to use it. The KELS was presented at two conferences, one of which was the National American Occupational Therapy Association Conference in 1979. After that time, many occupational therapists across the nation began to use the KELS with success. It has since continued to be distributed across the country and is taught by many occupational therapy schools.

Although the KELS was originally designed to be used in psychiatric settings, it has applicability to many patient populations. It is particularly effective with geriatric patients in acute care settings to assist with discharge planning. Rehabilitation units are also using the KELS with a variety of patient diagnoses. Other patient populations for which the KELS is an effective measure are the mentally retarded and special adolescent programs. In some states, the KELS is being used as an effective tool to assist in determining gravely disabled or involuntary treatment court cases. As health care has continued to move toward shorter hospital length of stays and as our geriatric population continues to increase, the Kohlman Evaluation of Living Skills has become more applicable to a variety of settings and populations.

Review of the Literature

The identification of an individual's performance in activities of daily living and the enhancement of that performance to optimal levels are the focus of occupational therapy intervention. Occupational therapists are involved with the successful integration of an individual into the natural environment[1] and with providing the individual with as much productive participation in society as possible.[2] Since the deinstitutionalization trend of the 1960s and 1970s, treatment in mental health settings is increasingly concerned with the integration of the mentally ill into the community as productive members.

The ability to perform is a factor which often causes patients to seek psychiatric treatment. Patients or relatives present the problem in terms of an inability to do that which was once done, or that which is necessary within the environment. Being able to work, study, rest, play, and care for is one of the barometers used to identify mental illness and health.[3]

There is an intrinsic need to deal with the environment.[4] As an individual learns to interact effectively with the environment, competence is increased. The individual learns about his relationship with the environment which creates a feeling of efficacy and satisfaction. Motivation is conceived to involve the satisfaction that occurs in successful experiences with the environment.[4] Motivation and satisfaction are barometers of mental health.

Activities of daily living are all methods in which an individual interacts and controls the environment. If an individual is unable to function and adapt to the environment, imbalances in work, self care and leisure activities occur, then competence, satisfaction, and motivation decrease and the individual's health is impaired or threatened. In many health care settings today, the integration of patients into the community is frequently a component of care plans. This is particularly true of chronic mentally ill patients who frequently change living situations and have difficulties adapting to the environment.

Occupational therapists have the skills to identify the level of function in daily living skills and to facilitate successful performance and integration of individuals into the community. If a patient is placed in a living situation and has difficulty performing the necessary basic living skills for that situation, further stress is added to the individual's tenuous adjustment and this actively interferes with integration into the community.[5] There is a need to place individuals in living situations that match the ability to perform daily living skills in order to increase the possibility of successful integration into the community.[6]

Occupational therapists have used informal assessment procedures since the inception of the profession.[7] In the 1960s, occupational therapists began to be concerned about developing formal assessments. There was an increasing concern with obtaining baseline data from which to plan interventions.[7]

In the area of living skills, there was no standardized evaluation that met the needs of a short-term psychiatric setting in determining the levels of function. The most commonly known evaluation of living skills for psychiatric patients is the Comprehensive Evaluation of Basic Living Skills.[8] The authors identify it as an eight-hour evaluation that is not intended for use with acute clients, in crisis intervention, or in short-term psychiatric facilities.[8] It is also an unstandardized evaluation. The Functional Life Scale is another living skill evaluation, but not developed by occupational therapists.[9] It also is a lengthy evaluation for long-term patients and doesn't meet the needs of occupational therapists in short-term settings.

The Independent Living Skills Evaluation[10] is directed at evaluating clients in a semi-supervised apartment living program. It takes 2½ hours to administer and does not have reliability and validity data. Another living skill evaluation is the Community Living Skills Assessment Inventory[10] which focuses on institutionalized handicapped individuals and includes many items related to physical disabilities. These items are not appropriate for psychiatric patients, and the evaluation is too detailed and lengthy for use in short-term care.

In gerontology there are some living skill evaluations, but none adequately meet the needs of psychiatric patients. Some of these are the Geriatric Functional Rating Scale,[11] the Functional Activities Questionnaire,[12] the Functional Assessment Inventory,[13] and the Self-Evaluation of Life Function.[14] The evaluation that most meets the needs of psychiatric patients is the Geriatric Functional Rating Scale,[11] which is designed to determine the need for institutional care. Its limitations are that it is based only on a self-report interview with very limited items of a global nature.

Frequently, mentally ill patients will use several health care facilities, both inpatient and outpatient. In this process, continuity of care is difficult to maintain and repetition of care can occur. Donaldson stated that most rehabilitation facilities have an ADL evaluation form, but there is no one such form that is widely accepted and used.[15] This situation is true in most mental health facilities with living skill evaluations. There has been a need for a unified standardized evaluation that has applicability to many settings. A unified evaluation more objectively measures change, increases communication between therapists, professions, and facilities and decreases repetition in patient care.

Administration

The Kohlman Evaluation of Living Skills assesses 18 living skills categorized under five main areas. These areas include: 1) Self Care, 2) Safety and Health, 3) Money Management, 4) Transportation and Telephone, and 5) Work and Leisure. Interview and task performance procedures are used to evaluate the living skills. In the administration section of the manual, the necessary equipment, the administration, and the specific scoring criteria for each section are given. Separate descriptions for scoring and equipment are also included in the manual. Examples of completed KELS score sheets are located at the back of the manual.

Instructions are included for assembling the list of equipment, such as a bar of soap, a bill, and local phone number cards. Four pictures to be used in the Safety and Health section are included in the manual and are essential in the accurate administration and scoring of the KELS. Other necessary supplies are local telephone books and a telephone. All of the equipment and forms, except for the telephone supplies, will fit in a three-ring binder so that it is easily transportable. The forms are included in the manual and may be copied if intact and the copyright is retained on the form. The scoring sheet is designed so that it may be copied onto standard progress note paper, if applicable for the setting. All the questions, tasks, and supplies are designed to simulate the local environment of the patient.

In the administration section of the manual, specific instructions are given for each item. These include how to present the equipment and the statements to be made by the evaluator. These must be stated as given, and feedback regarding the patient's performance should not be made until the end. The instructions are to be followed precisely or the results may not be valid or reliable.

Scoring

Independent and Needs Assistance are the scoring categories for the KELS. Specific scoring criteria are given with each section of the evaluation. The scoring criteria are designed to indicate the minimum standards required to live independently in the community. Independent is defined as the level of competency required to perform the basic living skill in a manner that maintains the safety and health of the individual without direct assistance of other people.[16]

For special situations in which the patient does not score within the scoring criteria given, the terms Not Applicable and See Note are used. These terms should be used as infrequently as possible and explanations made on the KELS Scoring Sheet.

To score the results, each section marked Needs Assistance, excluding Work and Leisure, is counted as 1 point. Needs assistance scores under Work and Leisure are counted as only a half point. Independent, See Note, and Not Applicable are counted as 0 points. A score of 5½ or less indicates the patient is capable of living independently and a total score of 6 or more indicates the patient needs assistance to live in the community. On the KELS Score Sheet (Figure 8-1), the scores for each section are blackened in to facilitate ease in reading and comprehending the results. At the bottom of the KELS Score Sheet, a short summary note is written. In the summary, the overall results are discussed and recommendations for appropriate living situations are made. The need for further occupational therapy intervention is indicated in the note.

When giving the Kohlman Evaluation of Living Skills, additional information is obtained about the patient's skills and abilities. Although reading and writing are not scored, the evaluator is able to determine if the patient has these abilities. With the Safety and Health pictures, which are purposefully designed to be dark, the patient must have figure-ground skills to determine what is safe in the pictures. This skill is very important in ambulating safely and maintaining a safe environment.

Throughout the KELS, there are many opportunities to assess the patient's cognitive abilities such as memory, attention span, and comprehension. The evaluator also learns about the patient's judgment and if the patient is in touch with reality. In the Work and

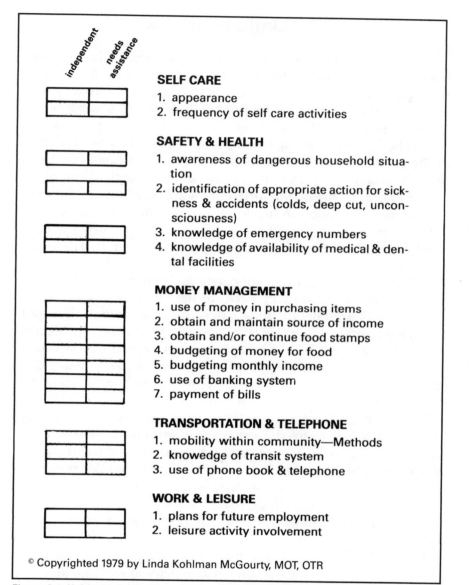

Figure 8-1. Kohlman Evaluation of Living Skills (KELS) score sheet.

Leisure sections, information about the patient's time use is obtained. This additional information gathered during the evaluation is not scored, but is tremendously valuable in making treatment plans with the patient. The important additional information should be included in the summary note at the bottom of the KELS Score Sheet.

Limitations

As with any assessment, the Kohlman Evaluation of Living Skills has its limitations and problems that may be encountered in administration and scoring. At times a patient will give a partial answer and the evaluator must ask additional questions to obtain a complete answer. Since this is a clinical decision-making process that cannot be controlled in the administration, there may be variations in the judgment of partial answers and the subsequent questions that are asked. Therefore, it is possible that a patient might be scored higher or lower by a different evaluator. More examination of potential differences in the administration process is needed.

One limitation of the KELS is that in order to keep the total administration and scoring time at a practical and short length, some items are knowledge based versus performance based. Therefore, in some cases, the occupational therapist may not be confident that the patient will actually perform the living skill, even if the knowledge is present. In those cases, the occupational therapist may need to do additional performance-based assessments beyond the scope of the KELS. Occupational therapists are strongly encouraged to regard the KELS as just one of many living skill evaluations. Supplemental evaluations need to be completed at the discretion of the individual evaluator.

If the KELS is going to be used in an occupational therapy program, it is helpful to educate other professionals how to evaluate the items and how to interpret and use the results. Without education, misinterpretation of results can occur. Education by a variety of means, such as individual contacts, written materials, and in-services, may be effective. Periodic re-education of staff is important to maintain the communication and understanding regarding the KELS.

Another problem in the administration and scoring is that some evaluators feel that to be normal a patient should score all items in the Independent category. The term Needs Assistance should not be viewed as being abnormal or negative. Many people function very independently in the community and receive some assistance in daily living skills. An example is the housewife whose husband manages the money. The housewife would probably score Needs Assistance for Obtain and Maintain Source of Income and Budgeting of Monthly Income. In the overall score, the housewife may function independently, but at present, needs assistance in those areas.[16] The KELS was not designed with the intent that Independent be scored in all areas. The circumstances and daily living environment of the patient must be considered.

It is also important to recognize that the KELS is an evaluation that is rarely, if ever, used as the sole determinant of a patient's living situation. The KELS is used to provide specific information regarding a person's ability to function in basic living skills. This information is only one aspect of the decision-making process of a multidisciplinary treatment team in determining discharge plans with a patient. The KELS is not meant to be used alone, but as a valuable, contributing factor in assisting the team to make discharge plans that will allow the patient to function as independently as possible in the community.

Research

By 1987, six research studies were completed. All were done on relatively small samples, but have helped to establish the reliability and validity of the KELS. In order to document the effectiveness of the Kohlman Evaluation of Living Skills, more extensive research using larger sample sizes and examining more variables is needed.

An interrater reliability study was completed in 1981 by Ilika and Hoffman[17] in Minnesota. This was an unpublished study in which the authors reported that the interrater correlations were significant at $p \leq .001$ with a variance from 74% to 94% agreement. The study involved psychiatric patients; the exact research design is unknown. Since this study, minor changes have been made in the administration and the percent of agreement for reliability was higher in later studies.

Ilika and Hoffman[18] also completed a concurrent validity study in 1981. This study was also unpublished and was conducted in a psychiatric treatment setting. The KELS score was compared to the Global Assessment Scale scores. Results indicated correlations of .78 to .89 with significance at $p \leq .001$. These results were favorable since both tests examine dysfunction in psychiatric patients, but evaluate different factors.

In 1982, Kaufman[19] completed a concurrent validity study. This study with psychiatric inpatients compared scores on the KELS with scores on the Bay Area Functional Performance Evaluation (BaFPE). The total BaFPE test score correlated with the KELS test score at $-.84$ ($p \leq .0001$). The negative value is a result of the test scores varying in opposite directions. These results contributed to establishing the validity of the KELS because both tests are designed to evaluate function and dysfunction in psychiatric patients, but do evaluate different indicators.

Tateichi[20] also completed a concurrent validity study in 1984. This study compared 20 subjects living in a halfway house (CCF) and 20 living independently (N = 40). The primary hypothesis was that clients living independently are more likely to have lower scores on the KELS than clients living in a sheltered setting. A low score on the KELS indicates greater independence. When the scores were compared using the Mann-Whitney U Test, results were significant (U = 47, p ≤ .001), with subjects living alone scoring lower on the KELS than subjects living in the sheltered setting. Tateichi also looked at whether the cut-off score of 5 differentiated between the two groups. Unfortunately, a score of 5½ should have been used to be consistent with the administration instructions. According to the results, the cut-off score of 5 was statistically significant, (p ≤ .05), but with a high incidence of false negatives. In this study, a false negative occurred when a person scored more independent in living skills (i.e., less than 5) than the setting required. Of the clients living in the sheltered setting, 45% scored greater than 6 and were accurately identified, while 55% scored less than 5. This could be expected because people live in halfway houses for a variety of reasons. A deficiency in living skills is only one possible reason. Of the clients living alone, 90% scored less than 5 and were accurately identified, while 10% scored greater than 6.

There is concern for this 10% of the clients who scored greater than 6 and who were, in fact, living alone in the community. In order to determine problems with the KELS, it would be important to analyze other variables between the two groups (the 90% and the 10%). For instance, what assistance were the clients receiving, how long had each client been living alone, was each client still living alone four to six months later, and what was the hospitalization rate? Without additional information, it is difficult to know if the KELS needs changes to be more valid. Prior to the testing in the study, interrater reliability was established on three consecutive trials, with the percentages of agreement at 84%, 94%, and 94%.

In 1985, Morrow[21] completed a predictive validity study. The KELS was administered to 20 inpatients on a geriatric unit. These pre-discharge KELS scores were compared to actual living situations 40 to 60 days after hospital discharge to determine if the KELS could accurately predict placement. Thirteen subjects were discharged to community living and seven subjects were discharged to nursing homes. A community support scale was designed as a supplemental scoring scale to the KELS. If a patient scored a Needs Assistance on an item in the KELS, the community support scale defined specifically what assistance the patient needed to remain in the community, and an adjusted KELS score was calculated. In predicting which geriatric individuals would succeed in community placements 40 to 60 days post-discharge, both the KELS and the adjusted KELS scores were 100% accurate. For those individuals with KELS scores greater that 5½ who had been recommended for nursing home placement, 50% were actually living in the community. Using the adjusted KELS score improved the positive predictive value to 72% with this group.

One problem with this study's interpretation is that nursing home placement is not recommended for all patients scoring greater than 5½. The KELS cut-off score of 5½ actually means that an individual with a score greater than 5½ would need assistance in order to live in the community. The community support scale did create a systematic scoring method to help the occupational therapist determine the kind of assistance needed in order to remain in a community living setting. This community support scale could be of great help in quantifying the assistance needed and in reducing discharge planning time for the treatment team. The community support scale is being strongly considered for inclusion in a revised edition of the Kohlman Evaluation of Living Skills. Interrater reliability was calculated on two consecutive trials prior to the study, and 100% agreement was achieved in scoring the KELS and the adjusted KELS.

In 1987, McGourty completed a predictive validity study. The purpose of the study was to determine if the KELS could predict successful independent living 40 to 60 days after discharge from the hospital. The subjects were 50 psychiatric inpatients who were discharged to live alone in the community. Each subject was administered the KELS in the hospital and the treatment team that made disposition plans were not given the results. Forty to 60 days after discharge, a follow-up contact was made to determine if the subject was still living independently. The percent of agreement calculated for interrater reliability was 98%. The validity results were much less favorable.

Several major problems were identified in the research design after data collection. One was the extreme variance in the size of the two groups. Two patients scored greater than 5½, and 44 scored 5½ or less (predicted to live alone). Therefore, very few patients who were predicted not to have the necessary living skills to live alone were discharged.EP The staff of the treatment teams had been using the KELS to assist with discharge planning for over two years. It was felt that the occupational therapists during those two years had been very effective in educating the staff to look for critical factors for successful independent living. Therefore, the staff did an excellent job in discharging patients to live alone who would have scored well on the KELS (5½ or less). This created an unexpected problem for the research study in that not enough patients scored greater than 5½. In the future, it is recommended that the staff not be familiar with the KELS prior to a study.

Another problem was in the follow-up contact. Nineteen patients were not living alone 40 to 60 days after discharge from the hospital. The study did not have a method to sort out legitimate reasons for not living alone. Only the yes-no response was analyzed. With the data, it could not be adequately determined if the patient was not living alone due to the failure to perform living skills or some other valid reason. In some cases, roommates moved in or the patient went to a residential mental health program, either of which could have had nothing to do with living skills. For many of the patients, no reason was identified. Because of the extreme limitations found in the research design, the results were disappointing. In the future, some of the problems in the research design could be eliminated.

Suggested Further Research

The research studies completed as of early 1987 have all contributed to making the Kohlman Evaluation of Living Skills an effective evaluation tool. Further research is needed in order to establish more completely the reliability and validity of the KELS. Larger sample sizes, broader geographical representation, and greater variety in research design are needed. Some suggestions for further research are:

1. Interrater reliability—Multiple observers score videotapes of the KELS being administered.

2. Consistency in administration—Comparison of groups learning the KELS by the manual only versus the manual and videotape instruction.

3. Predictive validity—Studies using a variety of populations and time frames to determine how accurately the KELS predicts over time and what other factors affect success in community living.

4. Concurrent validity—Studies in a variety of settings with many

populations to examine if patterns of living skills occur with specific populations and settings. Additional studies with large sample sizes and geographical representation administering the KELS and collecting demographic data with chronic psychiatric patients living alone.

These are only a few of the many possible research projects that are needed. More studies investigating the validity of the KELS are necessary, but are difficult to design. Isolating living skills as the only changing variable can be very challenging, particularly over an extended period of time. This is especially true when the patient populations tend to lead very unstable lives. Even though the research designs may be difficult, the studies are needed in order to give occupational therapists a living skill evaluation that is even more reliable and valid.

Summary

The Kohlman Evaluation of Living Skills is a valuable assessment tool for occupational therapists. Research has been conducted on the validity and reliability, although more studies are needed. The KELS is an effective measure in assisting the occupational therapist to determine the living skills of a patient and whether a patient can live alone. With the current health care trends of shortened hospital stays and community living, an evaluation of this nature is critical. The Kohlman Evaluation of Living Skills is an assessment that can be used in a variety of settings with many patient populations. It can be given in a short period of time and the administration procedures can be learned easily. The Kohlman Evaluation of Living Skills is an essential assessment tool for occupational therapists and occupational therapy programs.

References
1. Johnson TP, Vinncombe BJ, and Merrill GW (1980). The independent living skills evaluation. Occupational Therapy in Mental Health 1, 5-17.
2. Black BJ and Chapple ED (1981). Rehabilitation through productive participation: Still waiting in the wings? Psychological Quarterly 53, 85-92.
3. Overview of OT in Mental Health. (1981). Unpublished. American Occupational Therapy Association, 1-17.
4. White RW (1959). Motivation reconsidered: The concept of competence. Psychological Review 66, 297-333.

5. Broekema MC, Danze KH, and Schloemer CU (1975). Occupational therapy in a community aftercare program. Am J Occup Ther 29, 22-27.

6. Gauger AB, Brownell WM, Russell WW, and Retter RW (1964). Evaluation of levels of subsistence. Archives of Physical Medicine 45, 286-292.

7. Diasio K and Moyer E (1980). On psychosocial assessment. Occupational Therapy in Mental Health 1, 1-3.

8. Casanova JS and Ferber J (1976). Comprehensive evaluation of basic living skills. Am J Occup Ther 30, 101-105.

9. Sarno JE, Sarno MT, and Levita E (1973). The functional life scale. Archives of Physical Medicine 54, 214-220.

10. Switzky HN, Rotatori AF (1978) Community living skills assessment inventory: An instrument to facilitate deinstitutionalization of the severely developmentally disabled. Psychological Reports 43, 1335-1342.

11. Graver H and Birnbom BA (1975). A geriatric functional rating scale to determine the need for institutional care. Journal of the American Geriatric Society 23, 472-476.

12. Pfeiffer E, Johnson TM, and Chiofolio RL (1981). Functional assessment of elderly subjects in four service settings. Journal of the American Geriatric Society 29, 433-437.

13. Cairl RD, Pfeiffer E, Keller DM, Burke H, and Samis HV (1983). An evaluation of the reliability and validity of the functional assessment inventory. Journal of the American Geriatric Society 31, 607-612.

14. Linn MW, and Linn BS (1984). Self-evaluation of life function (SELF) scale: A short comprehensive self-report of health for elderly adults. Journal of the American Geriatric Society 39, 603-612.

15. Donaldson SW et al (1973). A unified ADL evaluation form. Archives of Physical Medicine 54, 175-179.

16. McGourty LK (1979). Kohlman Evaluation of Living Skills, KELS Research.

17. Ilika J and Hoffman NG (1981). Reliability study on the Kohlman evaluation of living skills. (Unpublished).

18. Ilika J and Hoffman NG (1981). Concurrent validity study on the Kohlman evaluation of living skills and the global assessment scale. (Unpublished).

19. Kaufman L (1982). Concurrent Validity Study on the Kohlman Evaluation of Living Skills and the Bay Area Functional Performance Evaluation. Master's thesis, University of Florida.

CHAPTER 9

THE MILWAUKEE EVALUATION OF DAILY LIVING SKILLS (MEDLS)

Carol A. Leonardelli, MS, OTR

Although occupational therapists have been treating the daily living skills of the mentally ill since the beginnings of the profession,[1,2] the process for determining the level of these skills has often been relegated to informal observation, report by nursing staff, or self-report by clients. When occupational therapists use assessments with specific procedures and methods for eliciting daily living skills data, the assessments usually were developed for a unique population or program at a particular hospital or facility and had little applicability to a broader mentally ill population. The Milwaukee Evaluation of Daily Living Skills (MEDLS), the assessment described in this chapter, was developed out of a desire to provide a measure of the behavioral performance of the daily living skills of long-term psychiatric clients which 1) would include standard administrative procedures and specific criteria to determine level of function, and 2) could be used for that population regardless of location.

Historical Development

Development of the MEDLS is based on measurement theory as described by Benson and Clark[15] and supported by Hemphill.[17] Benson and Clark suggest that instrument development follow a step-by-step, four-phase process of planning, construction, quantitative evaluation, and validation. Hemphill proposes several criteria that should be considered to determine if an evaluation is appropriate for a specific use. These include reporting of a rationale for developing the instrument, description of the population for whom it was designed, use of measurable behaviors, clear administration procedures, reports on norms, validity and reliability, and guidelines for interpretation of results.[16] The MEDLS was designed to meet these criteria, following the four-phase process described by Benson and Clark.

The planning phase initially involved identifying the purpose, target group, content area of the instrument, and review of the literature as described. The next part of planning was the identification of experts in the area of psychiatric occupational therapy and daily living skills. Six experts were identified and enlisted to serve as consultants to the project.

The experts were asked to respond to a questionnaire regarding functional areas of daily living skills for the chronically mentally ill.

This included a rank ordering of a list of skills and indication if the skill was best measured by self-report, demonstration of performance, or actual performance.

The experts were also asked to respond to several open-ended questions regarding evaluation of daily living skills. These questions included a critique of other evaluations for daily living skills currently available, consideration of a feasible amount of time for evaluation administration, the relative value of using Uniform Terminology for Reporting Occupational Therapy Services as developed by the American Occupational Therapy Association (AOTA) in the evaluation instrument, and the appropriateness of a proposed operational definition of the target population.

Responses from the experts were analyzed and interpreted. The following objectives were established for the evaluation instrument:

1. It will assess behavioral performance in the skill areas of basic communication, medication management, personal care and hygiene, time awareness, dressing, eating, personal health care, safety in the home, use of telephone, use of transportation.

2. It will have standard administration procedures.

3. It will use performance of skill as compared to self-report when feasible.

4. It will be developed with independent units or subtests so administration can be individualized and it is feasible to use relative to time.

5. It will use terminology that is clear and understandable to all mental health disciplines.

With objectives identified, the planning phase was completed. The construction phase began with item development. Items to elicit actual performance of skills were written in clear and understandable terminology following a uniform format and in a manner that would differentiate levels of function. An equipment list, screening form, and reporting form were also written.

This first edition of the MEDLS was then reviewed by the expert consultants and 73 occupational therapists across the country to establish content validity. Based on input from the clinicians and expert consultants, several items on the MEDLS were revised and new subtests in maintenance of clothing, safety in the community, and use of money were developed. This revision concluded the construction phase of development and resulted in the present Research Edition of the MEDLS.

The third phase of development is quantitative evaluation. This involves a pilot administration, reliability studies, and revision of the instrument as necessary. This phase is currently underway.

The final phase of validation, particularly predictive validation, will be conducted at a future date.

Review of the Literature

Rationale for the Development of the MEDLS

As the literature in psychiatry continues to support the concept of "deinstitutionalization" as a more humane and cost-effective way of treating the chronically mentally ill in our society,[3,4] alternatives to long-term residence in mental hospitals are still being sought. Accurate means of assessing an individual's potential to live in these less structured settings need to be developed. The ability to perform necessary basic living skills was identified as one of six factors crucial to a client's success in functioning under less supervision or in the community.[4] The ability of the occupational therapist to accurately and reliably determine a client's level of performance in daily living skills is a necessary component of successful efforts of deinstitutionalization in psychiatric practice.

There have been six evaluations of daily living skills published in the occupational therapy literature, specifically designed for psychiatric clients.[2,5-9] Four of these instruments are not appropriate for use with the institutionalized chronically mentally ill as indicated by their designation for use in acute care settings, their use of self-report, which is considered unreliable for chronic psychiatric clients,[10] the exclusion of skill areas that may be critical to thorough assessment or their structure as screening devices. Three of the four instruments do not report any research on validity or reliability. The Scorable Self Care Evaluation by Clark and Peters reports reliability and normative data.[7]

Of the two remaining daily living skills evaluations for psychiatric clients described in the occupational therapy literature, both are specifically designed for a chronically mentally ill population.[8,9] The Independent Living Skills Evaluation assesses daily living skills necessary for an apartment living program in the community.[8] It is completed by the therapist, based on observations and subjective judgments of the client's abilities and potentials. The client also completes the evaluation as a self-admininstered questionnaire. There are no reports of research on the instrument's validity and reliability, nor can it be interpreted for less independent living situations, such as group homes, or for totally independent community living. The authors are to be commended for the comprehensiveness of the instrument and the detailed descriptors for scoring. The Comprehensive Evaluation of Basic Living Skills is more appropriate for determining a wide range of abilities and potential living situations. However, it is extremely long, lacks any validity or reliability data, and does not consistently use uniform administration procedures.[9]

Behavioral Performance as a Measure of Function

The focus of the MEDLS is assessment of the behaviors/skills needed for adequate functioning in the client's anticipated living situation (expected environment). The pathology causing the lack of those behaviors or interfering with performance is not addressed. This approach is acceptable and consistent with applied behavioral research and behavioral assessment.[11,12] However, when behavioral performance is used as a measure of function and pathology is not specifically addressed in an assessment instrument, the following questions must be considered by the evaluator:

1. What constitutes effective performance of the behavior for the individual being evaluated?

2. How does the individual's performance deviate?

3. What interfering behaviors exist?

4. Under what circumstances is the desired performance to be maintained?

The format and structure of the MEDLS attempt to address some of these issues, but certain judgments always will be left to the discretion of the evaluator. For example, each subtest of the MEDLS has several skills that need to be performed in order for the client to receive the maximum score. Although an effort was made to isolate specific behaviors which can be defined and measured, the qualitative performance and evaluation of such skills as "expresses self clearly" or "maintains suitable posture" will vary from client to client and evaluator to evaluator. The decision as to whether or not the quality of performance will be *effective for an individual client* will always rest with the professional evaluator.

The presence of other factors interfering with adequate performance of skills is a common problem with the chronically mentally ill. Clinicians who reviewed this instrument during its development indicated repeatedly that clients may be able to perform the stated skills, but might be unwilling or unmotivated to do so. Other factors that may interfere with actual performance of skills include disorientation, limited attention span, hostility, passivity, poor impulse control, limited organizational skills, poor problem-solving abilities, and so on. It does not seem feasible to evaluate and measure these dysfunctional behaviors as part of an evaluation of daily living skills. These factors must be identified under "Comments" on the Reporting Form and their presence considered in the interpretation of the results of the MEDLS. The need to consider these other behaviors, or characteristics of the client, implies the importance of multi-dimensional assessment of the client. The MEDLS should be considered as only one component of the total evaluation. Its limitations as a measure of behavioral performance must be recognized.

The impact that the client's expected environment or potential discharge placement has on evaluation and treatment cannot be overemphasized. It is a poor use of time and resources, and useless to the client, to focus treatment on maintenance of clothing and living space when the client is going to a skilled nursing facility where these services are most likely provided.

Unfortunately, a client's expected environment is often not known until shortly before discharge and simply may be dictated by the availability of bed space elsewhere. Clinicians often have no reliable means of identifying what skills are most significant to an individual client. Each subtest of the MEDLS is a separate, independent unit that is administered and scored autonomously. A wide range of tasks is included from self-care and hygiene to use of transportation and first aid. This provides more flexibility to the evaluator in selecting subtests to meet a client's needs and the potential demands of the expected environment.

A final aspect to consider when using behavioral performance as a measure of the client's ability to function, is the relative value of self-report by the client. As stated previously, the limitations of behavioral performance must be recognized in a thorough evaluation of the client. Self-report may need to be used in some areas of evaluation where behavioral performance might be too intrusive (e.g., toileting) or impractical (e.g., use of transportation).

The limitations of self-report as a valid means of determining the abilities of the chronically mentally ill was articulated repeatedly by occupational therapists who reviewed the MEDLS during its development. There was a consensus by these clinicians, when asked about the preference of "performance of skill" as compared to self-report, that "performance of skill" was the only valid means of determining if a chronically mentally ill client was able to do a task. As one clinician reported, "clients often deny difficulties in skills until they are actually asked to perform them." The use of self-report has been kept to a minimum in the MEDLS. Some skill areas may not seem to be addressed as thoroughly in an effort to avoid asking the client "how" they would do something, for example, "frequency of self care."

Individual Versus Group Measurement

The evaluation of an individual's performance, whether it be in the area of daily living skills or any other realm of intervention appropriate to occupational therapy, is essential in documenting therapeutic accountability. The MEDLS is designed to measure individual client performance and provide baseline data for treatment. It includes 21 subtests which can be used individually or in any combination for a specific client (reliability and validity are being determined for each subtest). It has many of the attributes considered necessary in an instrument designed to measure the status of an individual as described by Kane and Kane.[13] These attributes include the ability to detect problems amenable to intervention, the ability to document increments of change to measure progress, and a sound methodology for sampling the behaviors measured.

However, the real value of the MEDLS, or any measure of functional living skills of the chronically mentally ill, may be in its ability to determine the potential future placement of an individual client. What daily living skills are necessary to function in a halfway house as compared to a community-based residential facility? What is the "normal" level of functional living skills in a group home? Can the MEDLS serve as a measure of performance of different groups of the chronically mentally ill living in settings with varying degrees of structure and supervision?

Measures of groups of individuals must meet the same requirements of reliability and validity as individual measures, with an emphasis on interrater reliability. Kane and Kane[13] identify other desirable attributes of group measures including the ability to distinguish broad categories of functional ability, ease of administration relative to time and cost, and decreased dependence on professional judgment of evaluators.

The differences between group and individual measures are not necessarily absolute differences, but may be degrees of relative emphasis.[13] Traditionally, assessments in the behavioral sciences have focused on comparison between an individual and a norm group, or between groups in various performance categories.[14] Can the MEDLS, an instrument designed to measure an individual's performance, serve as a measure of that person's performance as compared to a particular group of chronically mentally ill? Probably not. However, the same skill areas need to be considered for the individual or group measure. To allow for comparison, another version of the MEDLS may need to be developed to serve as a group measure if no suitable measure is currently available.

Clientele

The population for whom the MEDLS was developed includes the types of residents still found in large psychiatric institutional settings across the country, skilled nursing facilities, community-based residential facilities, halfway houses, group homes, and those individuals attending outpatient or day-treatment programs while functioning marginally in the community. This type of client is operationally defined as an adult, age 18 years old and above, with a history of mental illness of at least two years duration, who has been hospitalized or under care at a skilled nursing facility for a cumulative period of at least six months within the past two years, or receiving weekly outpatient treatment due to mental or emotional disorder for a minimum of two years.

Administration of the MEDLS

The MEDLS has four major components: a screening form, equipment list, subtests with administration procedures and appendices, and a reporting form. Each component will be discussed separately.

Screening Form

Through use of the Screening Form, it can be determined in what skill areas a client needs to be evaluated. The evaluator decides which subtests to use based on information from the medical record (nursing notes, admission note, etc.), input from other health care personnel and family, initial observations and interview, and professional judgment. The Screening Form serves as a quick reference for the evaluator and others as to which skill areas need to be evaluated and in which the client is independent (see Appendix D). A "Not known at this time" column is provided for use when the evaluator does not have enough information on which to decide the client's status. A mark in this column should serve as a "red light" to the evaluator that this item needs to be re-examined when the evaluator is more familiar with the client.

Equipment List

The equipment list of the MEDLS is divided by subtest. Some equipment is used in more than one subtest; this overlap is indicated on the equipment list so duplicate equipment need not be acquired. The client may provide his own equipment in such areas as dressing and personal care. All equipment should consist of normal consumer products, rather than institutional products.

Subtests

The MEDLS consists of 21 subtests. More may be added with future revisions of the instrument. The subtests are designed to be used individually or in any combination, according to the client's needs. Each subtest is scored separately according to the number of subskills needed to be effectively completed for competence in the skill area. Level of performance in each subtest is indicated by a score measured in relation to the overall score for that subtest alone.

Each subtest follows the same format (see Appendix E). Listed for each are the method to be used, equipment needed, procedures to elicit performance, list of skills to be performed, maximum time allowed to perform skills, and scoring criteria. If the client is unable to complete the skill within the time limitations, the evaluator must use professional judgment to determine if the client has a deficit in performance ability, comprehension of expectations, motivation, or if there are other interfering factors. The evaluator will *determine the score based on the performance* and address the other areas under "Comments" on the Reporting Form.

The MEDLS is not suitable for administration in a group format. Group testing of skill performance permits mimicking of behaviors among group members and does not elicit individual abilities.

Behaviors Assessed. Basic Communication Skills: These skills are evaluated throughout the assessment. Several subtests are used involving verbal interaction or a task activity group for a period of 30 to 40 minutes. The subtest addresses responsive and expressive abilities.

Dressing: These skills are evaluated by two methods. The first is actual performance of ability to dress within 10 minutes. It is recommended that the evaluator observe the client actually dressing in the morning, rather than observing a simulation at another time in the day. An interview is conducted to determine the client's judgment of suitable clothing for certain weather conditions and activities.

Eating: Eating skills are assessed by evaluator observation while the client is eating a meal. Skills evaluated include posture, handling of utensils, interaction with others, and judgment on food quantities.

Maintenance of Clothing: This subtest requires the client to demonstrate ability to launder, dry, and fold clothing, and sew a button on a shirt.

Medication Management: The client's ability to use prescribed medications effectively is assessed by a structured interview and a review of the medical record. The interview assesses the client's understanding of his need for medication, its side effects, knowledge of his medication schedule, and judgment regarding renewing the prescription. The evaluator must be knowledgeable about the client's medication regimen, side effects, and so on. Review of the medical record assesses client compliance with the medication regimen. The evaluator must be aware that compliance within an institutional setting is no assurance that the client would follow through with medication if unsupervised. The "Comment" section could include remarks relative to dependency and attitude toward authority, which would influence compliance.

Personal Care and Hygiene: This section is divided into nine separate skill areas. None of the subtests addresses frequency of self-care tasks. This can only be evaluated by self-report, which is generally considered unreliable for this population.[10]

Toileting: These skills are assessed by a structured interview and medical record review. The interview addresses feminine hygiene which is not scored for males or post-menopausal females. It also asks the client to describe use of the toilet. The review of the medical record determines bowel and bladder control. The evaluator must be aware of any physical condition that would affect control.

Brushing Teeth: The ability to brush teeth is evaluated by observation of the client actually performing the task.

Denture Care: In this subtest, the client is asked to demonstrate how dentures are stored and cleaned.

Bathing: Bathing skills and safety are evaluated by a simulation of bathing or showering activities. The selection of bathing or showering is determined by availability and/or client choice.

Use of Make-up: The client is first asked if they use make-up. If the response is affirmative, she is instructed to apply the amount she would use. This subtest requires the evaluator to make a subjective judgment as to the culturally and socially acceptable amount of make-up the client should use. There is inherent bias in this subtest.

Shaving: This subtest can be used for women who shave their underarms and legs, and men who shave their face. The client has a choice between use of an electric or safety razor. Skills assessed include adequate hair removal and safe handling of razor.

Nail Care: The client is asked to trim and clean his fingernails and toenails with a nail clipper and clean up when finished.

Hair Care: The evaluator observes the client washing his hair. This should occur at a time when the client is in need of a shampoo.

The client is assessed on his ability to shampoo, rinse, dry, and comb his hair, and clean the sink area.

Eyeglass Care: The client is asked to demonstrate cleaning and storing his glasses. Clients are also asked to describe what they would do if their glasses were broken.

Personal Health Care: This subtest assesses the client's judgment in meeting his health care needs. An interview poses two questions regarding actions to take when feeling ill. The client is also asked to demonstrate application of medicine and bandage to a "wound."

Safety in Community: This subtest uses an interview and diagrams to evaluate a client's judgment regarding crossing streets, locking doors, use of sidewalks, and hitchhiking. Because of the impracticality of assessing actual performance of these skills, the subtest relies on self-report.

Safety in Home: To assess clients' judgment in functioning safely in their places of residence, they are asked to simulate an emergency phone call and respond to interview questions. The interview uses diagrams depicting unsafe household equipment and smoking in bed.

Time Awareness: As a measure of time awareness, the client is asked to read the time on traditional and digital clocks. The client is also asked to record or report his daily schedule of activities and use a bus or subway schedule. The evaluator then reviews the client's attendance in therapy, at meals, or at medication administrations for a designated period of time as an indicator of his responsibility to time commitments.

Use of Money: In this subtest, the client is asked to count money, make change, and select items equaling $10 or less from a Budget List.

Use of Telephone: To evaluate telephone skills, the client is asked to locate a number in the phone book and make a call from a pay telephone.

Use of Transportation: The ability to use transportation is assessed by an interview. The client is asked to describe how he would use public transportation and how he would access shopping facilities. It is impractical and unrealistic to assess actual performance; however, the reliability of the client's self-report needs to be considered.

Reporting Form

The Reporting Form of the MEDLS is designed to be included in a client's medical record (see Appendix F). In one page, the client's strengths and weaknesses in daily living skills are recorded.

Scoring. Each subtest is scored separately based on the total sub-skills for that area. There is no cumulative score for the MEDLS. Level of performance in each subtest is indicated by a score measured in relation to the overall score for that subtest alone. Deficits in specific skills are indicated by using "key words" in conjunction with the score for that skill area. The "key words" are included in the administrative procedures for each subtest and are to be recorded directly on the Reporting Form. The Reporting Form indicates the skill and if a client is below maximum level of performance. A marking of "No Evaluation Needed" (NEN) is used if the skill is not relevant to the client (e.g., denture care) or if the client is known to be competent in that area. The form is designed to allow for reporting of a re-test of the MEDLS at a future date.

Suggestions for Future Research. Reliabiliy, validity, and normative studies are currently underway. Predictive validity studies are planned for the future. The author would encourage others to participate in the ongoing development, validation, and improvement of the MEDLS when the manual becomes available.

Summary

The MEDLS is designed to provide baseline data for establishing treatment objectives for an individual patient. It should be used to guide treatment. Use of the scoring format provides quantifiable measure of change. This type of information is invaluable in providing data on accountability and cost effectiveness to third party payors and hospital administrators. The MEDLS includes screening and reporting forms which provide quick, easy-to-read information to the entire treatment team, and a comprehensive equipment list divided by subtest.

The MEDLS is a measurement of client performance of skills. Self-report by clients has been kept to a minimum. It has been used only when performance of skills was unrealistic because of the personal nature of the skill (e.g., toileting) or impractical because of time limitations (e.g., use of transportation).

It is strongly recommended that the "Comments" section of the Reporting Form be used to identify behavioral problems of the client which may impede task performance. Issues such as dependency, motivation, and hostility are not specifically addressed in the MEDLS, but need to be considered in any skill performance.

There are some daily living skills not included in the MEDLS which may be appropriate to the client. Although more subtests may be added and current subtests further developed, users are urged to identify other evaluations of daily living skills currently available.

References
1. Hopkins HL and Smith HD (1983). Willard and Spackman's Occupational Therapy (6th ed). Philadelphia: Lippincott.
2. Mosey AC (1973). Activities Therapy. New York: Raven Press.
3. Beard JH, Propst R, and Malamud, TJ (1982). The Fountain House model of psychiatric rehabilitation. Psychosocial Rehabilitation Journal 5, 48-50.
4. Stein LI and Test MA (1980). Alternative to mental hospital treatment. Archives of General Psychiatry 37, 392-399.
5. McGourty LK. Kohlman Evaluation of Living Skills (2nd ed). Seattle: KELS Research.
6. Broeckema MC, Danz KH, and Schloemer CU (19 75). Occupational therapy in a community aftercare program. Am J Occup Ther 29, 22-27.
7. Clark EN and Peters M (1984). Scorable Self-care Evaluation. Thorofare, New Jersey: Slack.
8. Johnson TP, Vinnicombe BJ, and Merrill GW (1980). The independent living skills evaluation. Occupational Therapy in Mental Health 1, 5-18.
9. Casanova J and Ferber J (1976). The comprehensive evaluation of basic living skills. Am J Occup Ther 30, 143-147.
10. Glazer W, Sholomskas D, Williams,D, and Weissman M (1982). Chronic schizophrenics in the community: Are they able to report their social adjustment? American Journal of Orthopsychiatry 52, 166-171.
11. Baer DM, Wolf MM, and Risley TR (1968). Some current dimensions of applied behavior analysis. Journal of Applied Behavior Analysis 1, 91-97.
12. Hawkins RP (1979). The function of assessment: Implications for selection and development of services for assessing repertoires in clinical, educational and other settings. Journal of Applied Behavior Analysis 12, 501-516.
13. Kane RA, and Kane RL (1981). Assessing the Elderly. Massachusetts: The Rand Corporation.
14. Ottenbacher K (May 25, 1984). Personal correspondence.
15. Benson J and Clark F (1982). A guide for instrument development and validation. Am J Occup Ther 36, 789-800.
16. Hemphill BJ (1982). The Evaluative Process in Psychiatric Occupational Therapy. Thorofare, New Jersey: Slack.

CHAPTER 10

FUNCTIONAL ASSESSMENTS USED WITH OLDER ADULTS

Betty Risteen Hasselkus, PhD, OTR
Gail Hills Maguire, PhD, OTR

Since the year 1900, the proportion of people in the United States 65 years old and older rose from 4% to 12%; the absolute number increased from 3.1 million to 28.0 million. This older population itself is getting older with the largest increases occurring by far in those aged 85 or older. This differential growth within the aging population is resulting in greater proportions of people at the extremes of old age.[1,2]

Although older people comprise only 12% of the total U.S. population, they occupy at least 30% of hospital beds and account for one fourth of all drug expenditures. The percentage of older people in institutions (primarily nursing homes) increases dramatically with age, reaching a high of 23% for persons over age 85 in 1980. At any one point in time only 5% of people over age 65 are in institutions, yet an estimated 39% will experience a stay in an institution some time before death.[3]

Among the community-living older population, most persons have at least one chronic condition. The need for functional assistance with activities of daily living increases sharply with age, with an estimated 46% of persons 85 years or older needing the assistance of another person to perform one or more personal or home management activities.[1] Ellis[4] referred to these aging population trends as the "demographic imperative," stating that occupational therapists must "respond by identifying and addressing critical issues in aging" in all spheres of professional activity.

Health in Old Age

Health in old age is a complex, elusive concept. Older people are subject to multiple diagnoses of both chronic and acute disease. At the same time, the elderly are experiencing normal developmental age changes such as gradual changes in endurance, vision, hearing, and reflex timing. Some problems in old age are due to long-time disuse or misuse of physical and mental abilities: back problems may occur because of lifelong postural habits or long use of a sagging mattress; or a new widow may struggle for the first time to make independent decisions regarding home maintenance.

Finally, traumatic injury may occur such as a hip fracture or cerebral vascular accident. In such an incident, it must be remembered that the trauma, whether it be primarily physical or psychological, occurs in conjunction with chronic and acute disease, normal age changes, and changes due to misuse or disuse. Snow and Rogers[5] describe this complex combination of normal and pathological changes in old age as a "delicate balance" of adaptation. "Incidents, which on the surface appear trivial, may serve to create dangerous imbalances in ... older adults" (p. 352). Treatment is aimed at maintaining the balance, preventing imbalances, and re-establishing the balance.

The multi-dimensionality of health in old age is reflected in current trends toward multi-dimensional assessment instruments and Geriatric Evaluation Units (GEUs). The interrelatedness of physical, mental, and social factors mandates this multi-dimensionality, but, since there is no general agreement in the aging literature concerning the content of such assessments, there is considerable variation among instruments. Rubenstein[6] reported that most multi-dimensional assessments include physical health, functional ability, psychologic health, and social parameters.

As Kane and Kane[7] suggest, the tools that health providers use to assess the needs of older people help to shape their views of the reality of older people. These authors state that measures of functional ability are the most useful overall indicators of health in old age. Older patients "are not diseased objects but people with families who live in communities and who view their health needs in the larger context of their social structure and personal life" (p. 133). Evaluations of the elderly must be administered and interpreted within the context of their normal life situations.

The systematic assessment of functional capacity is the core concept of occupational therapy in gerontology. However, just as there is no universal agreement as to what constitutes a multi-dimensional assessment of the aged, so too is there little agreement as to what constitutes a functional assessment of the aged in occupational therapy. Therapists may develop informal clinical evaluation tools, may select from among several uni-dimensional instruments, may utilize all or part of a test battery such as the OARS Methodology,[8] or use a combination of these tools. In many cases standardized instruments are not available for all aspects of the multi-dimensional or functional assessment, and therefore the validity and reliability of the instruments cannot be established. The multi-dimensionality of health in old age, that is, the "delicate balance" of adaptation in the elderly, creates in the therapist the dilemma of paradoxically trying to use or develop standardized evaluation techniques for a population of people who require exquisitely fine-tuned individualized approaches in treatment. Somehow, psychometrically sound yet holistic approaches to assessment must be developed.

Functional Assessments Used in Occupational Therapy

For the purposes of this discussion, functional capacity is defined as the ability to perform specific daily living tasks which are normally expected of an individual within a social environment.[9] While the concept of functional capacity and its measurement emerged several decades ago in connection with workmen's compensation benefits, its relevance to an understanding of health in old age was increasingly recognized in the 1960s.

Physical Self-Maintenance Scale and Instrumental Activities of Daily Living Scale

In 1969, Lawton and Brody[10] published an article detailing the development of two scales to measure function in older people—the Physical Self-Maintenance Scale (PSMS) and the Instrumental Activities of Daily Living Scale (IADL). Within Lawton's schema of competence, the scales represent measures of two levels of function, with the IADL requiring greater neuropsychological organization than the PSMS. Within each level, the complexity of activity is also arranged hierarchically. For example, the PSMS measures the lowest level life maintenance tasks of toileting, feeding, dressing, grooming, mobility, and bathing; a 5-point Likert-type scale of performance for each task was developed, ranging from complete independence to complete dependence. The IADL scale focuses on activities that Lawton conceptualized as the next higher level of function, that is, using the telephone, shopping, food preparation, housekeeping, laundry, transportation, medication management, and finance handling. Each of these tasks is also hierarchically scored based on degree of independence. Lawton and Brody's scales have been cited and utilized extensively in gerontological literature as valid and reliable measures of function in older people.

One example of the use of the PSMS and IADL in treatment planning and research is the study reported by Rubenstein, Josephson, Wieland, et al.[11] in which the effectiveness of a Geriatric Evaluation Unit (GEU) was systematically assessed. An occupational therapist was a member of that evaluation unit which was designed to provide improved diagnostic assessment, therapy, rehabilitation, and placement. The PSMS and IADL scales were used in conjunction with a morale scale and a mental status scale to measure function in GEU and control groups at baseline, 6-month and 12-month time periods. Improvement in function was significantly greater in the GEU group than the control group.

From the author's own earlier work on the PSMS and the IADL, as well as work by other investigators, Lawton developed the Multilevel Assessments Instrument (MAI), which has also been used widely by a variety of gerontology professionals.[12]

Barthel Self-Care Index

Another widely used scale to measure basic functional ability in the elderly is the Barthel Self-Care Index.[13] Originally designed as a measure of function in the physically impaired, it has been used extensively in research and treatment planning with older people. Hasselkus[14] described the use of the Barthel Self-Care Index with a population of geriatric home care patients. The index measures basic self-care skills of feeding, transfer, personal hygiene, toileting, bathing, ambulation, stairs, dressing, and bowel and bladder continence. Scoring is based on observation of performance, and preferential weighting has been given to items of continence and mobility. Hasselkus[14] used the Barthel Index in four ways: to help define the amount and type of personal care services required by patients to be maintained in the community; to document change over time (the scale was administered every six months); to better define variables associated with discharge/placement decisions; and to help clarify the impact of community health services on the ability of the family to maintain care of an older member over a long period of time.

Parachek Geriatric Behavior Rating Scale

The Parachek Geriatric Behavior Rating Scale[15] is a quick screening device of 10 multiple-choice items. Three questions on physical condition, four on general self-care, and three on social behaviors are included. Each question is scored on a 5-point Likert-type scale of performance, with 1 being the most impaired. The final score is the sum of the 10 individual ratings. The Parachek Scale was derived from the longer Plutchik Geriatric Rating Scale.[16] Cutting scores predicted placement of 74.5% of the geriatric patients tested.

A treatment manual has been designed for use in conjunction with the Parachek Scale. Scores on the scale are divided into three levels. Group I are patients scoring in the 10-to 24-point range. Descriptions of possible occupational therapy treatments include positioning, sensory stimulation, motor patterns, and group process. Treatment suggestions for group II patients scoring in the 25- to 39-point range include self-care activities, more advanced sensory stimulation and group activities, contact with the community, and adaptation for wheelchair patients. The highest functioning group with scores between 40 and 50 can manage most self-care activities and may be candidates for placement in a community setting. Treatment suggestions for patients in this group include opportunities for control over their lives. The rationale for grouping patients according to their functional levels is that it makes it easier and more cost effective to provide appropriate programs.[16]

Short Portable Mental Status Questionnaire

The Short Portable Mental Status Questionnaire (SPMSQ) is another screening device which is used extensively by physicians and other health personnel to detect intellectual impairment.[17] While it is a myth that most older adults eventually experience some form of dementia, nevertheless 11% to 12% of the U.S. population over age 65 has a mild to moderate dementia and 5% has a severe dementia which precludes independent living. The proportion increases as age increases, and at least 50% of all nursing home clients are there because of dementias.[18]

The 10 questions on the SPMSQ include such items as what is the date today, what is your telephone number, who is the president of the U.S. today, and subtract 3 from 20 and keep subtracting 3 from each new number. Three or four errors indicate a borderline deficit, and five or more errors indicate a moderate to severe impairment. Adjustments in scoring are made downward (subtract one point) for college-educated persons and upward (add one point) for those with less than a high school education. The SPMSQ is intended to be a quick screening tool for cognitive dysfunction. It has been used to predict reliability of response to functional assessment tools.[19] Snow,[20] in a review of mental status assessment in older people, described other mental status tools which the author felt were more useful for treatment planning in occupational therapy, in particular the FROMAJE[21] and the Set Test.[22]

New Instruments Developed by Occupational Therapists

Recently, occupational therapists have begun to develop instruments which measure functional capacity for use in therapeutic treatment planning for the elderly. The examples of occupational therapy instruments which are described in this chapter reflect both institutional and community contexts; represent preventive, maintenance, and restorative treatment goals; and are aimed at both the well elderly and the impaired. Both the older individual and the environment are addressed.

There is an acknowledged need for occupational therapy assessments which empirically demonstrate reliability and validity.[23-28] This is especially true in assessment of the elderly where the multi-dimensionality of health in old age mandates more complex multi-dimensional measurement instruments.

Assessment of Occupational Functioning

The Assessment of Occupational Functioning (AOF)[23] is an occupational screening device based on the model of human occupation. It is a semi-structured interview schedule to assess physically and psychologically impaired residents in long-term treatment settings. The AOF is divided into six components including: values, personal causation, interests, roles, habits, and skills.

After obtaining the information on the interview, the therapist rates each of the six areas on a 5-point Likert scale of descriptors, with a rating of 1 being the highest level of functioning and 5 being the lowest level. A total score between 6 and 30 may be obtained by adding the scores of the six components. Disappointing results on an initial sample of 83 community and institutionalized elderly subjects suggest minimal estimations of reliability and concurrent validity, and low ability to discriminate between healthy and institutional adults.[23] The authors cite limitations of the study which include the raters' knowledge of subject assignment by group, and the mixed results of comparison with the Geriatric Rating Scale by Plutchik.[16] The authors conclude that further research is needed.[23]

Performance Assessment Self-Care Skills (PASS)

Focusing broadly on functional assessment and the elderly, Rogers[29] is developing an instrument which is designed to provide a systematic overview of the older adult's task performance in activities of daily living. The Performance Assessment of Self-Care Skills (PASS) contains items which represent self-care and instrumental tasks that are relevant to independent living, and that can be carried out in the clinic or the home under natural or simulated conditions.

Scoring. Scoring on the PASS is competency-based and takes into account the task itself and the teaching approach that facilitates the older person's best performance. For example, the test item in which the client is instructed to "Show me how you make your bed" is scored on the following dimensions: goal attained, safety, adequacy, nature of the impairment, level of independence, frequency of help, nature of help, equipment, and completion time. The "nature of the impairment" covers a wide range of mental and physical factors such as limited muscular strength, postural imbalance, inattention, and memory deficit. So too the "nature of help" includes such items as emotional support, visual guidance, and physical assistance. This scoring system provides information to the therapist on potential therapeutic interventions as well as self-care status.

In addition to the 35 performance test items for personal and instrumental tasks, the PASS contains three behavioral items. Spoken Language Ability and Comprehension of Spoken Language are each scored on a global rating scale that ranges from "no problem" to "severe." The third behavior item, Frustration Tolerance, is scored on a scale of 1 to 5 according to the level of frustration that is displayed during the performance tasks.

Standardization. Administration and scoring of the performance task items are standardized by the following instructions on the instrument: 1. the task is named, 2. the conditions under which the task is to be performed are described, 3. the behavior needed to complete the task is described, 4. the standard for the task accomplishment is defined, and 5. the instructions to be used are given. Alternate conditions for in-hospital use (vs. in-home use) are provided. For example, within the activity "Dressing," the following protocol is given:

Task: Don outer clothing appropriate for wearing on a cold and rainy day.

Condition: Home setting—no special preparation.

Behavior: Locate outer wear; put on selected clothing; remove clothing.

Standard: Selection of a heavy raincoat or sweater and raincoat; a rainhat or umbrella.

Instructions: "Dress as you would to go outside on a cold and rainy day."

Condition (in-hospital): Given a selection of in and outdoor clothing.

Instructions: "Here is a selection of clothing. Dress as you would to go outside on a cold and rainy day."

Rogers views content validity as the most important validity estimation for a criterion-related instrument such as the PASS. Content validity of this instrument is derived from three commonly used geriatric instruments upon which the PASS items were based.[8,10,30] An initial list of performance test items was developed and then reviewed by a panel of two occupational therapists, one nurse, and two neuropsychologists, all of whom are specialists in geriatric practice. The final test items on the PASS were the result of this process. Rogers plans to collect normative data on a sample of normal elderly and also to establish test-retest reliability.

Tri-level ADL Assessment

Maguire's Tri-level ADL Assessment[31] organizes activities of daily living into the six categories of communication, food needs, dressing, hygiene, mobility, and organization. Tasks in these categories are followed through the three environmental levels of personal, home or sheltered environment, and the community. This enables the therapist and elderly person to identify not only specific tasks, but also the environmental area(s) which are most problematic in order to determine how to help maintain independence. The scoring method (which may be revised) is a modification of the system used by Iverson[32] for the Revised Kenny Self-Care Evaluation. In the first step of the scoring, each item is assigned a rating from independent to dependent. Secondly, a quantitative rating is assigned to each of the three environmental levels of each category.

The Tri-level ADL Assessment represents an attempt to organize ADL measurements in a comprehensive manner. No validity or reliability estimations have yet been done.

Assessment of Home Safety of Well Elderly

A home safety awareness survey (self-report) developed by Buchanan[33] assesses awareness of more than 100 safety aspects of the home environment. For example, kitchen safety aspects include lighting, electrical wiring, ventilation, and flooring. A score of 0 represents the safe environment where the factors that cause accidents would be at a minimum. The highest possible raw score is 145, indicating the most dangerous environment, with factors that cause accidents being at a maximum.

The author also has developed a safety training program including a slide/tape presentation to educate elderly persons on safety in the home. Buchanan pre-tested and post-tested the training program, using the safety awareness survey with a small number of well female clients between 70 and 80 years of age. After completion of the safety training program, clients' awareness of potential dangers that existed in their homes increased by 9%.

Medication Management Functional Assessment Tool

The elderly in this country are major consumers of prescription and non-prescription drugs. Approximately 40% of these older drug users are dependent on medication to be able to pursue desired and necessary activities of daily living.

Recognizing the importance of medication usage in the lives of so many older people, Rajek and Smith[34] developed a Medication Management Functional Assessment Tool. "The ability to functionally manage self-administration of prescription medications is often dependent upon an individual's emotional, cognitive and physical skills, environmental expectations, and existing or available support systems" (Medication Management Functional Assessment Protocol). The multi-dimensionality of this otherwise seemingly discrete daily living skill is immediately apparent.

In the medication management tool, knowledge of the medications (name, dose, expected action, side effects, etc.) is combined with actual task performance assessment such as locating medications, opening containers, and bringing medication to the mouth. In conjunction with the task performance, the older person is asked "How do you remember when to take your medication(s)?" This question yields information on what unique cueing techniques the individual utilizes which can then be used to help develop effective and meaningful adaptations to enhance the medication management. Cues are categorized as being primarily visual, written, auditory, cognitive, assistance from others, space or location specific, or tactile. The assessor is advised not to consider unconventionality of a personal system as "wrong" or in need of change unless the system puts the older person at risk for adverse side effects or injury.

The Medication Management Functional Assessment Tool is still in the development stage. In piloting the instrument, the occupational therapists found evidence of such factors as item redundancy (e.g., having separate questions about special instructions *and* special precautions), inappropriateness (asking about expiration date rather than refill date), and the difficulty in clarifying the question about side effects without simultaneously giving verbal cues or gestures which led to biased responses. The information on personal cueing methods proved to be particularly useful for understanding existing management strategies and for planning mutually satisfying adaptations. A standardized form of the medication management tool is being developed for future use in therapeutic program planning as well as research.

Summary

This brief overview of functional assessments used with older adults is not meant to be inclusive of all available formal and informal instruments developed by occupational therapists or others. It is a sampling of tools which demonstrate the complex issues facing occupational therapy in assessment of the elderly.

There is presently no clear definition of the areas which constitute a functional assessment nor a comprehensive instrument. Therefore, the therapist needs to carefully identify the scope and parameters of each client assessment, not just for the purposes of research, but also for treatment planning and when entering the assessment results into the medical record.

Occupational therapy is in a state of growth and development in assessment. A number of occupational therapy tools are being developed or refined based on specific models of therapy and designed for particular populations. If, as Kane and Kane[7] suggest, the tools that are used by health professionals help to shape their views of the reality of older people, then occupational therapists perhaps deserve some credit for historically recognizing a reality which is appropriately multi-dimensional and complex. Now it is time to develop increased sophistication in the area of assessment so that the occupational therapy profession may mature in developing practice skills based on defined theory and documented by sound research which represents valid and reliable measurement.

References

1. American Association of Retired Persons (1985). A Profile of Older Americans: 1985. Washington, D.C.
2. Soldo, BJ (1980). America's elderly in the 1980s. Population Bulletin 35(4). Washington D.C.: Population Reference Bureau, Inc.
3. Vicente L and Wiley JA (1979). The risk of institutionalization before death. Gerontologist 19, 361-367.
4. Ellis NB (1985). Aging: Occupational therapy and the demographic imperative. Occupational Therapy Newspaper, 39(5).
5. Snow TJ and Rogers JC (1985). Dysfunctional older adults, in Kielhofner G (ed): The Model of Human Occupation: Theory and Application. Baltimore: Williams and Wilkins, 352-370.

6. Rubenstein L (1983). The clinical effectiveness of multi-dimensional geriatric assessment. Journal of the American Geriatrics Society 12, 758-762.
7. Kane RA and Kane RL (1981). Assessing the Elderly: A Practical Guide to Measurement. Lexington, Kentucky: Heath.
8. Pfeiffer E (ed) (1976). Multidimensional Functional Assessment: The OARS Methodology. Durham, North Carolina: Duke University, Center for the Study of Aging.
9. Functional Limitations: A State of the Art Review (1978). Falls Church, Virginia: Indices, Inc.
10. Lawton MP and Brody E (1969). Assessment of older people: Self-maintaining and instrumental activities of daily living. Gerontologist 9, 179-186.
11. Rubenstein LZ, Josephson KR, Wieland GD, et al (1984). Effectiveness of a geriatric evaluation unit. The New England Journal of Medicine 311, 1664-1670.
12. Lawton MP, Moss M, Fulcomer M, et al (1982). A research and service oriented multilevel assessment instrument. Journal of Gerontology 37, 91-99.
13. Mahoney F and Barthel D (1965). Functional evaluations: The Barthel index. Maryland State Medical Journal 14, 61-65.
14. Hasselkus, BR (1982). Barthel self-care index and geriatric home care patients. Physical & Occupational Therapy in Geriatrics 1(4): 11-22.
15. Miller ER and Parachek JF (1974). Validation and standardization of a goal-oriented, quick screening geriatric scale. Journal of the American Geriatrics Society 22, 278-283.
16. Plutchik R, Conte H, Lieberman M, et al (1970). Reliability and validity of a scale for assessing the functioning of geriatric patients. Journal of the American Geriatrics Society 18, 491-500.
17. Pfeiffer E (1975) A short portable mental status questionnaire for the assessment of organic brain deficit in elderly patients. Journal of the American Geriatrics Society 23, 433-444.
18. Schneck MR, Reisberg B, and Ferris SH (1982). An overview of current concepts of Alzheimer's disease. American Journal of Psychiatry 139, 165-173.
19. Pfeiffer E (1982). Functional assessment inventory. Tampa, Florida: Sun Coast Gerontology Center.
20. Snow T (1983). Assessing mental status. Gerontology Special Interest Section Newsletter 6(1): 1-3.

21. Libow L (1981). A rapidly administered, easily remembered mental status evaluation: FROMAJE, in Libow L and Sherman E (eds): The Core of Geriatric Medicine. St. Louis: Mosby, 85-91.

22. Isaacs B and Kinnie A (1973). The set test as an aid to the detection of dementia in old people. The British Journal of Psychiatry 123, 467-470.

23. Watts JH, Kielhofner G, Bauer DF, et al (1986). The assessment of occupational functioning: A screening tool for use in long-term care. Am J Occup Ther 40, 231-240.

24. Hemphill BJ (1983). Mental health evaluations in occupational therapy. Am J Occup Ther 34, 721-726.

25. Hemphill BJ (ed) (1982). The Evaluative Process in Psychiatric Occupational Therapy. Thorofare, New Jersey: Slack.

26. Diasio K and Moyer E (1980). Editorial on psychological assessment. Occupational Therapy in Mental Health 1, 1-3.

27. Continuing education needs (1983). Mental Health Special Interest Section Newsletter 6(2).

28. Reporting on research—AOTA/AOTF: Standardized evaluations (1983). Occupational Therapy Newsletter 37(7).

29. Rogers JC. The Performance Assessment Self-care Skills. Western Psychiatric Institute and Clinic, Pittsburgh (unpublished).

30. Gurland B, Kuriansky J, Sharpe L, et al (1977). The comprehensive assessment and referral evaluation (CARE)—rationale, development and reliability: Part II, factor analysis. International Journal of Aging and Human Development 8, 9-42.

31. Maguire GH (1985). Activities of daily living, in Lewis C (ed): Aging: The Health Care Challenge. Philadelphia: Davis.

32. Iverson IA, Silberberg NE, Stever RC et al (1973). The Revised Kenney Self-care Evaluation. Minneapolis: Sr. Kenney Institute.

33. Buchanan A (1986). A home safety awareness program for the well aged: A preventive approach. Gerontology Special Interest Section Newsletter 9, 2-4.

34. Rajek MJ and Smith RO (1987). Functional Assessment Tool for Medication Management. Paper presented at the Annual Conference of the American Occupational Therapy Association, Indianapolis, Indiana.

Bibliography

Buchanan A. Home Safety Awareness Program. Nollamara, Western Australia.

Lawton MP. Multilevel Assessment Instrument Manual. Philadelphia Geriatric Center, Philadelphia.

Miller ER and Parachek JF. Parachek Geriatric Behavior Rating Scale: Revised and Expanded Treatment Manual. Center for Neurodevelopmental Studies, Inc., Phoenix.

CHAPTER 11

PRE-VOCATIONAL ASSESSMENT IN MENTAL HEALTH

Cindee Quake Peterson, MA, OTR

The concepts of work, productivity, and activity are synonymous with the practice of occupational therapy. An individual's level of productivity often defines socioeconomic status, life style, and quality of leisure time. Society measures a person's worth by what goods and services are contributed. Work is considered so essential to most people's feelings of self-worth and self-esteem, that any interruption in work-related activities can seriously affect mental health.

This chapter will attempt to identify the pre-vocational evaluation process as it relates to the client in a psychiatric setting, and identify standardized, commercially available evaluation tools applicable to this population group. Before proceeding into the pre-vocational evaluation process, it is important to discuss work-related skills from a developmental continuum.

Formation of work-related skills is part of the developmental continuum that occurs along with learning self-maintenance and leisure pursuits in childhood. Children acquire work-related behaviors and habits by observing role models in the home and school, and participating in environments where productivity is rewarded. A 2-year-old child learns to respect authority figures and discovers that compliance with parents' wishes brings about a positive form of feedback. Children entering the school environment learn that timeliness and punctuality are important habits, as are adhering to rules and regulations.[1,2] Developmental delay in obtaining work-related skills can occur due to mental retardation, mental illness, chronic disabilities, or environmental deprivation. Table 11-1 illustrates the developmental sequence and age equivalent that the average child performs work-related tasks.[3]

The individual with emotional, intellectual, or physical impairments is often considered job handicapped and has difficulty obtaining employment. The role of the occupational therapist in the pre-vocational evaluation process is to determine if the client has potential for employment, and assess whether the client needs to redevelop former work skills, or learn new behaviors and skills.[4] The client who requires redevelopment of former work skills may have lost a work-identity due to traumatic injury or a debilitating condition. The person who needs to learn new behaviors and skills may have never developed a work identity or role due to intermittent hospitalization or institutionalization.

Table 11-1
Developmental Sequence of Work-Related Skills

Age Equivalent	Activity
3-7 years	1. Elevating parent expectation of vocational potential of child. 2. Sorting (large cue difference) 3. Stacking 4. Attending behavior 5. Simple direction following
7-12 years	1. Working alone 2. Working in small groups 3. Higher rates of attending 4. Sorting (small cue differences) 5. Small assembly (hand and simple tool) 6. Switching task on command 7. Starting to work on time 8. Remaining at activity site until given permission to move
12-18 years	1. High rate of production of assigned task 2. High rate of attention on high or low interest tasks 3. Low error rate 4. High rate of switch-task compliance 5. Starting to work on time 6. Returning from breaks promptly 7. Remaining at work station 8. Signaling supervisor when encountering difficulties 9. Working alone 10. Working in groups 11. Working quietly 12. Recognizing work deficits 13. Correcting work deficits 14. Using common tools 15. Work site safety behavior

Source: Lynch, Kevin P., Prevocational and Vocational Education for Special Needs Youth. Brookes Publishing Co., Baltimore, 1982.

The client with psychosocial dysfunction often experiences hidden deficits that affect his chances of obtaining employment. Work habits, behaviors, and interpersonal skills often limit employability, rather than task performance and motor skills.[5]

Having considered the developmental level of the individual, the next procedure is the pre-vocational evaluation process described in Figure 11-1.[6]

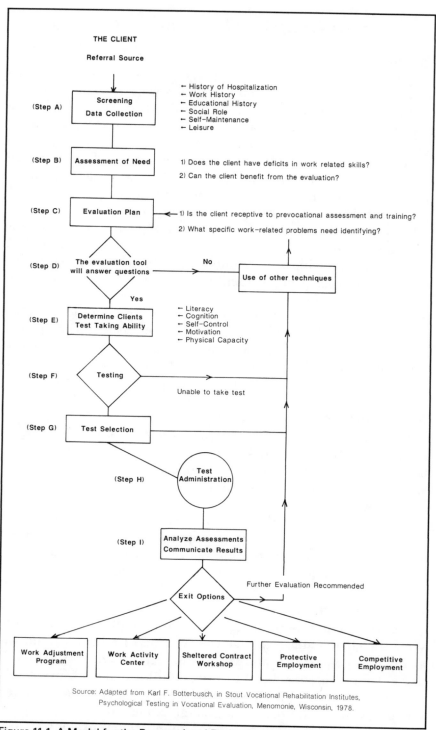

Figure 11-1. A Model for the Prevocational Evaluation Process.

The Pre-Vocational Evaluation Process

Screening

The occupational therapist collects data during the initial interview to obtain information on the client's work history, history of hospitalization, education, and social role (Step A). The therapist assesses whether the client can benefit from a pre-vocational evaluation. Does the client have identifiable deficits in the occupational performance areas of self-maintenance, leisure, and work-related skills (Step B). A client who demonstrates poor personal hygiene, or has a history of dependency regarding activities of daily living, will have difficulty securing and maintaining employment.

It should be determined if the client is receptive to pre-vocational assessment and training at this stage of the evaluation (Step C). A client who is receiving a government-subsidized income may not be motivated to receive employment training or assistance because of lack of perceived incentives for employment. The next question to ask in the pre-vocational evaluation process is whether the client has a realistic idea of his abilities, values, and interests regarding potential occupations. The screening will assist in determining which evaluations should be administered, the attitude and personal adjustment of the client, and functional performance skills.

Evaluation Plan

To determine vocational readiness, the occupational therapist should identify specific work-related problems in performance and skill areas through formal and informal assessment. The skills outlined in Table 11-2 contribute to successful and satisfying employment.[7,8]

Following identification of the client's problems with work-related skills, the therapist selects appropriate tests to determine if the suspected areas of deficit are valid. Will the test help ascertain the client's work-related problems (Step D, Table 11-2)

Test Appropriateness

When selecting methods of evaluation, the therapist must consider the client's ability to take the test (Step E). Literacy and the ability to follow written and verbal instructions are essential skills needed for written tests or to provide information through self-report. Many interest/preference checklists and behavioral and personality surveys require a sixth grade reading level.[9]

The therapist should observe for an emotional reaction to testing, including anxiety level, frustration tolerance, and the client's

Table 11-2
Essential Work-Related Skills

Cognitive/Learning Abilities

Reading level
Communication — Written and Oral
Ability to follow written and oral instructions
Decision making
Problem solving
Judgment
Memory — Auditory and Visual
Conceptual skills — Time concepts
                            Money concepts
                            Safety concepts

Perceptual

Figure-ground discrimination
Body scheme
Motor planning

Physical capacity

Dexterity — bi-manual, unilateral, fingertip
Speed of response
Eye-hand coordination
Endurance
Mobility
Strength
Sensation

Intrapersonal

Attitude
Self-awareness
Realistic identification of interests, abilities, values
Coping skills — ability to perform under time constraints

Interpersonal

Cooperation with co-workers
Ability to accept and respond to supervision

Work Habits

Punctuality
The ability to adjust to rules, regulations, and expectations
Concern for quality of work
Attending to task
Appearance and hygiene

motivation to perform at maximum potential. Test results can be easily sabotaged by the uninterested client. The client's ability to physically engage in the requirements of the test should be considered. An example would be the introduction of a test that requires bilateral motor activity to an individual with the use of only one arm. The client with psychosocial dysfunction often uses psychotropic medications that can impair test-taking ability. If the client is unable to respond appropriately to the test situation, he exits the evaluation process (Step F). The therapist either modifies the technique for obtaining information at this point, or a new evaluation plan is agreed upon by the therapist and client. The therapist needs to go back to Step D in the pre-vocational evaluation process.

Test Selection

The occupational therapist has been limited in selecting an evaluation tool for the psychiatric population group by the scarcity of standardized tools available that measure the behavioral and personal adjustment factors essential for successful employment. Therapists traditionally have relied on non-standardized, criterion-referenced test samples based on what a client can do. Unfortunately, third party payers only reimburse for services that have measurable data related to work potential and placement.[10] The occupational therapist must rely on standardized assessment measures in addition to informal testing because in the future, pre-vocational evaluation may become part of the Prospective Payment System for Medicare reimbursement of services in inpatient psychiatric settings. No evaluation tool should be used alone as a single predictor of potential, unless it is designed to measure all the skill areas and has demonstrated validity and reliability with a psychiatric population group. To the author's knowledge, no such tool has been developed (Step G). The following work-related evaluation tools are commercially available and are applicable to the client with psychosocial dysfunction.

Manual Dexterity. Among the most commonly used commercial tests in the pre-vocational evaluation process are the "Manual Dexterity" evaluations that measure speed and accuracy of motor coordination (Table 11-3). These evaluations are highly specific and should be selected according to how closely the test item resembles the job in question.[11] Test objectives must be met by providing realistic simulations of actual job-related requirements. The occupational therapist who develops well-constructed job samples may often find higher validities than demonstrated by commercially available tests. These tests primarily address the physical capacity of clients, an area in which psychiatric clients are not particularly impaired. Therefore, the tests have limited value in assessing the vocational potential of the emotionally impaired individual.

Interests, Preferences, Attitudes, and Values Surveys. Interest inventories are designed to measure a person's likes and dislikes for a variety of activities, objects, or personality types encountered in daily living. Interest surveys are valuable assessment tools in determining personal preference regarding types of vocations and also illustrate whether the client has a realistic concept of the skills needed to perform various occupations.[11] The unskilled client who wants to become a major-league baseball player may not have the necessary self-awareness to make an appropriate choice regarding occupation and will need assistance in determining realistic vocational goals (Table 11-3).

Aptitude Tests. Aptitude tests are used to measure an individual's status in a variety of abilities such as verbal, numerical, spatial visualization, and perceptual speed. Aptitude tests give a more accurate measure of a person's abilities than I.Q. tests because each trait is measured separately, and a client can score high in one area and low in another without negatively affecting the overall score.[11] Aptitude tests also give a profile of an individual's strengths and weaknesses. Aptitude tests have been traditionally administered by psychologists and educators, although occupational therapists would benefit from having access to the test results for goal setting. Occupational therapists have the skills to administer aptitude tests; some evaluations require special training. Most aptitude tests are machine scored with an interpretive printout of the test results (Table 11-3).

Behavioral and Personality Tests. Behavioral and personality tests measure emotional adjustment, interpersonal relations, motivations, and attitudinal characteristics. The tests are typically administered as self-report, situational, or as projective techniques.[11] Although psychological testing has been the domain of licensed psychologists, occupational therapists have developed tools such as the Bay Area Functional Performance Scale that has a Social Interaction Scale (Table 11-3). Projective tests such as the Azima, BH Battery, Goodman, and Shoemyen have been widely accepted by the occupational therapy profession.[12]

Table 11-3
Commercially Available Standardized Pre-Vocational Evaluations

MANUAL DEXTERITY TESTS

Test	What does it measure?	Population Group	Assets	Limitations
Valpar	Measures 18 different work samples independent of each other, derived from job analysis of specific occupations	General population and industrially injured workers. Norms are available for deaf persons.	Work samples are appealing to clients and are easily administered and scored.	Individual work samples range from $500 to $1,500. Valpar does not provide instructions on how to produce a comprehensive final report. There is minimal consideration of psychosocial aspects of employment.
McCarron-Dial Systems Publisher: Common Market Press	Basic work evaluation system including verbal, spatial, cognitive, sensory, motor, emotional and integration coping. A Street Survival Skills Questionnaire is also available.	Handicapped populations above the age 15 involved in prevocational training programs in school settings.	The McCarron-Dial has strong neuropsychological component.	Cost: $1,325.00
Bennet-Hand Tool Dexterity Test Available from: The Psychological Corporation.	These timed manual dexterity tools measure speed of response, fine motor coordination, and the use of small hand tools.	Industrial workers, male and female above the age of 18.	There is no reading required.	Specificity of motor function requires that the tests resemble the acutal job itself as closely as possible.
Purdue Pegboard Available from: Science Research Associates				
Crawford Small Parts Dexterity Tests Publisher: Stanford University Press				

Table 11-3 (continued)
Commercially Available Standarized Pre-Vocational Evaluations

INTERESTS, PREFERENCE AND ATTITUDE SURVEY

Test	What does it measure?	Population Group	Assets	Limitations
AAMD-Becker Reading-Free Vocational Interest Inventory CR-Full Experimental Version (1975) Publisher: American Association on Mental Deficiency	Indentifies occupational interests of mentally retarded individuals in occupations at the unskilled and semi-skilled levels.	Educable mentally retarded at the high school level.	The Pictorial test items require no reading or mastery of the English language.	There is limited information available on validity and reliability
Kuder Occupational Interest Survey (KOIS) (1975) Publisher: Science Research Associates	The KOIS assists in making occupational choices by identifying interests in relationship to various occupations.	High school, college students, and adults making vocational choices.	Occupational scales are available for individuals who are not interested in additional formal education.	The individual must be able to read at a sixth grade level. A person with visual impairment would have difficulty reading the test items.
Wide Range Interest-Opinion Test (WRIOT) (1972) Publisher: Guidance Associates of Delaware, Inc.	The WRIOT "was designed to cover as many areas and levels of human activity as possible." The Pictorial test items range from unskilled through professional level jobs.	The test manual has information on the administration of the WRIOT to mentally retarded, physically handicapped, and disadvantages individuals.	The Pictorial format allows for the test to be used with individuals with handicaps.	Lack of information on validity and reliability.
Strong Campbell Interest Inventory (SCII) Publisher: Stanford University press	The SCII was developed to assist college students determine interest in professional or semi-professional occupations.	College students	Sets a standard in which other interest inventories are judged.	College orientations. Requires familiarity with many occupations and advanced school subjects

Table 11-3 (continued)
Commercially Available Standardized Pre-Vocational Evaluations

BEHAVIOR PERSONALITY TESTS

Test	What does it measure?	Population Group	Assets	Limitations
Vocational Adaptation Rating Scale (VARS) Available through: Western Psychological Services	Maladaptive behaviors likely to occur in vocational settings. The six scales include verbal manners, communication skills, attendance and punctuality, interpersonal behavior, respect for rules, and personal hygiene.	Standardized on over 600 severely to mildly retarded adolescents and adults.	Well standardized.	Rater has to be familiar with the individual and be able to observe behavior in a work setting.
Sixteen Personality Factor Questionnaire (16PF) Available through: The Psychological Corporation	Primary personality traits such as assertiveness, emotional stability, self-sufficiency.	Varied norms on males and females 14-29, prison inmates, schizophrenics, and culturally disadvantaged males.	A low literate form is available.	Highly educated may find the test easy to fake.
Bay Area Function Performance Evaluation (BAFPE) Publisher: Consulting Psychology Press	Task-oriented abilities and social interaction skills.	Age 16 and over, mentally ill.	Well defined set of norms for the M.I. population.	

APTITUDE TESTS

Test	What does it measure?	Population Group	Assets	Limitations
General Aptitude Test Battery Available from: U.S. Employment Services	Vocational significant aptitudes in general learning ability; verbal, numerical, spatial perception; form, clerical perception; motor coordination; and manual dexterity.	Normative data on 4,000 general workers. Norms developed for ninth and tenth grade students.	Has been used effectively with emotionally disturbed, retarded, and deaf clients.	Sixth grade reading level required. Formal training in administration is required.

Test Administration (Step H)

In the prevocational evaluation process, the occupational therapist administers the test following standardized protocol and procedure and interprets the results accordingly. Before test administration, the therapist should ensure that any qualifications for administering the test have been met, such as certification or training. There are vocational evaluation systems and commercially available tests that require or recommend training with a duration anywhere from one day to one week.

Exit Options (Step I)

Following the interpretation of the test results, the occupational therapist is involved with reporting results to the client, other professionals or a health care delivery team. The occupational therapist is involved with making recommendations regarding appropriate programming, training, or job placement following the prevocational evaluation process. The results of the evaluation may be inconclusive, and further evaluation may be recommended. The client may be referred to several types of settings.[13]

Work Adjustment Programs—Work adjustment programs provide the least demanding employment level and emphasize activities of daily living and ways of improving or decreasing inadequate or inappropriate work behaviors. Interpersonal communication, motor skills, personal hygiene, criticism coping, decision making, and timeliness are typical areas of remediation for the client who has not acquired basic work-related skills.

Work Activity Centers—Work activity programs are designed to simulate actual jobs in unskilled to semi-skilled occupations. Clients may be involved with sorting, classifying, and assembling and disassembling various objects with simple hand tools. Production rate is often measured to determine level of performance compared to competitive industrial workers.

Sheltered Contract Workshops—In a sheltered workshop environment, clients are involved in completing various jobs contracted through industry. Workers are paid at minimum wage or less, which is a cost-effective way for industries to complete jobs requiring manual dexterity and allow for better use of employees' time. The contract workers benefit by being in a sheltered environment where rate of production is lower and can learn work-related skills without the stress of competitive employment.

Protective Employment—Protective employment involves a regular employment position in which a company takes an interest in assisting the marginal worker with his skills and problems. A worker who has been recently hospitalized may require part-time employment until he has the necessary coping skills to return full time.

Competitive Employment—Competitive employment requires the ability to secure a regular work position and maintain a production rate equal to other employees. Competitive employment is ideally the ultimate goal that the occupational therapist works toward with the client, as are independent living skills. Not all clients are able to achieve a competitive level of employment and would benefit from less demanding work-related environments.

Summary

The pre-vocational evaluation process of the psychiatric client poses problems for the occupational therapist because of the lack of appropriate standardized assessments. Many work-related standardized asssssments measure physical capacity rather than interpersonal and personal adjustment factors, which are better indicators of employability for the mentally ill. The occupational therapy profession is making strides in developing projective instruments and performance scales for the emotionally impaired, although normative data are lacking, which is crucial for credible documentation for third party payers.

References
1. Reed KL and Sanderson SR (1983). Concepts of Occupational Therapy. Baltimore: Williams and Wilkins.
2. Maurer P (1968). Prevocational activities and evaluation for the child and adolescent. Physical Therapy 48, 771-776.
3. Lynch KP, Kiernan WC and Stark JA (eds) (1982). Prevocational and Vocational Education for Special Needs Youth: A Blueprint for the 1980s. Baltimore: Paul H. Brookes.
4. American Occupational Therapy Association (ad hoc committee) (1980). The role of the occupational therapist in the vocational rehabilitation process: Official position paper. Am J Occup Ther 34, 881-883.
5. Watts FN (1976). Modification of the employment handicaps of psychiatric patients by behavioral methods. Am J Occup Ther 30, 487-490.
6. Botterbusch KF (1978). Psychological Testing in Vocational Evaluation. Menomonie, Wisconsin: Stout Vocational Rehabilitation Institute.
7. Ethridge DA (1968). Prevocational assessment of rehabilitation potential of psychiatric patients. Am J Occup Ther 22, 161-167.

8. Distefano MK and Pryer MW (1970). Vocational evaluation and successful placement of psychiatric clients in a vocational rehabilitation program. Am J Occup Ther 24, 205-207.
9. Buros OK (ed) (1938-1985). Mental measurement yearbooks. New Jersey: Gryphon Press.
10. Anderson AP (1985). Work potential evaluation in mental health. Am J Occup Ther 39, 659-663.
11. Anastasi A (1976). Psychological Testing. New York: Macmillan.
12. Hemphill BJ (ed) (1982). The Evaluative Process in Psychiatric Occupational Therapy. Thorofare, New Jersey: Slack.
13. Parnicky JJ and Agin D (1975). Pathways Toward Independence. Columbus: Ohio State University.

CHAPTER 12

WORK TOLERANCE SCREENING

Linda Ogden Niemeyer, OTR, CVE

Purpose

Within the last two decades, vocational rehabilitation has become increasingly complex, with a resulting lack of continuity and interplay between the composite services that make up the vocational rehabilitation process. Programs with names such as work preparation, vocational readiness, pre-vocational assessment, independent living, or vocational evaluation can be found in rehabilitation centers, schools, sheltered workshops, and free-standing vocational evaluation centers. Vocational rehabilitation is provided for some individuals in the private sector, and for others is a service provided by the state.

Some specialized programs for particular service area recipients for example, pre-vocational programs for developmentally disabled adolescents, splintered off and became relatively isolated. Transition from patient to worker often means transfer from one reimbursement/service delivery system to another, with resultant delays and paperwork. One group that has suffered particularly from this fragmentation and increased complexity in vocational rehabilitation has been the adult psychiatric population. Evaluation and treatment services provided by occupational therapists can often bridge the gap between the medical and vocational rehabilitation systems and can ease the transition from "patient" to "worker." One particularly important service gap concerns the need for reliable and valid work tolerance evaluations.

The method of work tolerance evaluation presented in this chapter was developed jointly by Leonard N. Matheson, PhD, and Linda Ogden-Niemeyer, OTR, CVE, at the Employment and Rehabilitation Institute of California. This is a practical approach that is flexible to provide for individualization of evaluation planning, yet allows for a structured evaluation and uses selected standardized evaluation tools that are available in the public domain. Although this evaluation method was originally developed for use in the industrial rehabilitation setting, it is equally applicable to the adult psychiatric population. Many psychiatric patients have prior injuries, especially involving the neck and lower back. In addition, many suffer from severe physical deconditioning brought on by weeks or months of inactivity. The emotional and monetary cost of embarking on a vocational plan that is physically inappropriate for the psychiatric patient can be great. Thorough and timely evaluation of physical tolerances prior to return to work helps identify and deal with what could be a significant obstacle to re-employment of a psychiatrically handicapped individual.

Definitions

Work Tolerance Screening is defined as "an intensive short-term (usually one-day) evaluation that focuses on major physical tolerance abilities related to musculoskeletal strength, endurance, speed, and flexibility."[1]

During this evaluation, selected structured physical demands of work are simulated in a controlled setting. The demonstrated responses to these work demands are observed and documented. This information is used by the rehabilitation professional(s) as part of the process of developing an appropriate vocational goal. For example, the information can be used to determine whether the evaluee can return to his usual and customary occupation or perform the physical demands of a new job that is being considered as part of a vocational plan. It also can be used to clarify the evaluee's physical capabilities prior to or during an intensive vocational exploration process.

Work tolerances are the observed and measured physical capabilities that affect competence to perform the physical demands of basic work tasks. These tolerances are measured in terms of the ability to sustain a work effort at a prescribed frequency over a given period of time. Factors that affect performance include strength, flexibility, energy reserve, the presence of pain or other limiting symptoms, and the presence of cognitive or psychological limitations. A list of all possible work tolerances would be as long and varied as all possible physical demands of work. Work tolerances that are commonly observed and measured include sitting, standing, reaching, crouching/kneeling/stooping, lifting/carrying, pushing/pulling, walking, climbing, handling, fingering, feeling, gripping, torquing, talking, listening, and seeing. Sustained work performance is called work capacity, or physical capacity, and is inferred based upon the gathered work tolerance data. Work capacity is described in terms of the ability to sustain a given work effort over a prolonged period of time, maintain a steady flow of production at an acceptable pace and acceptable level of quality, and to handle a certain amount of pressure.

Historical Development

Observation and measurement of work tolerances is not new to occupational therapy. The history of the profession is rich with examples of work-related programs that include work tolerance evaluation. These programs reached a peak of development in the 1950s.

One of the earlier programs developed during this era was the "work-evaluation" program of the Rochester Rehabilitation Center in New York.[2] After completing the physical restoration portion of rehabilitation, evaluees were placed in a workshop environment and presented with a variety of jobs that utilized industrial working conditions and normal, or non-handicapped, industrial standards. Performance over a period of three to six weeks was carefully observed and analyzed in terms of such factors as work habits, strength, tool handling, and dexterity to determine areas of potential employability. Vocational interests were formally evaluated only after work tolerances were relatively stable and well-defined.

A service called "pre-vocational evaluation" was offered in the 1950s at the Institute for the Crippled and Disabled, also in New York.[3] Participants were assigned tasks in a simulated work setting to determine if they could develop work habits, work tolerances, coordination, and productive speed to a level that would be acceptable for entry into vocational evaluation. Those who subsequently entered the vocational evaluation program underwent a comprehensive assessment of their assets and limitations with regard to work aptitudes and skills.

By the late 1950s the movement toward using more standardized vocational testing procedures was well-developed. The practice and profession of vocational evaluation came into being as a comprehensive assessment process that used standardized work samples and psychometric tests to determine vocational potential in terms of work aptitudes, interests, temperaments, and skills.[4] In response to this trend, more standardized and structured work tolerance assessments were developed and administered by occupational therapists. "Work tests"[5] were developed by Lillian Wegg, OTR, in conjunction with the rehabilitation team of the May T. Morrison Center for Rehabilitation in San Francisco. The work tests were prepared in kit form and designed to be realistic in order to measure as accurately as possible the evaluee's response to actual job demands. Each test kit contained a manual that included the test description and purpose, the physical demands of the tasks, the psychological factors to be considered, and detailed instructions regarding administration and scoring. They were standardized with normative data based on the performance of non-handicapped workers familiar with the job in a competitive employment setting. Although more than 80 test kits were developed, the 25 most commonly used work tests simulated job tasks in clerical and sales work, service work, skilled mechanical work, and semi-skilled to unskilled manual work.

The "physical capacities evaluation"[6] was developed at the Woodrow Wilson Rehabilitation Center in Fisherville, Virginia. This evaluation consisted of a battery of tests focusing on selected work tolerance areas, including muscle testing, depth perception, color vision, touch discrimination, sitting, standing, walking, pushing and pulling, lifting, carrying, crouching, stooping, reaching, balance, climbing, crawling, grasp and release, manipulation, and writing. Each test was highly structured, but not formally standardized with normative data. The information gathered was descriptive, and was used to match the evaluee to prospective jobs. Job matching was based on data regarding the minimum physical requirements for training and performance in a number of given job areas.

The developers of both the work tests and the physical capacities evaluation used the *Dictionary of Occupational Titles*,[7] also called the *D.O.T.*, to provide a suitable framework upon which to organize the structure of the evaluation. This allowed for division and selection of appropriate evaluation tools according to either the major job categories or major physical work demand factors. Following the evaluation, the *D.O.T.* then could be used to identify possible appropriate job matches for the evaluee.

During the next two decades, progress made by occupational therapists in the development of work tolerance evaluations slackened, as the bulk of the profession moved to embrace the medical model and to develop its professional role within rapidly growing physical rehabilitation centers. Participation of occupational therapists in work-related programs decreased markedly. The 1980s were marked by a reawakening of occupational therapists to the importance of involvement in work-related programs and the need to fill service gaps being created by the emergence of new markets.[8,9] Both physical therapists and occupational therapists have responded to this need.

Two Models For Assessment of Work Tolerance

The approach developed at the Employment and Rehabilitation Institute of California uses two models in order to provide work tolerance assessment for a wide variety of evaluees. The first, called the ERIC Work Tolerance Screening Battery (EWTS Battery), is an intensive short-term evaluation that focuses on selected major physical tolerance areas. The second, called the Comprehensive Work Tolerance Evaluation (CWTE), is a longer term evaluation that allows the evaluator to gather data regarding such factors as

Table 12-1
Sources of Availablity for Evaluation Tools Used in the
E.R.I.C. Work Tolerance Screening Battery

Evaluation Tool	Source	Approximate Cost
Crawford Small Parts Dexterity Test	Psychological Corporation 7555 Caldwell Avenue Chicago, IL 60648	$300.00
Bennett Hand Tool Dexterity Test		$300.00
Minnesota Rate of Manipulation Test	CTB/McGraw-Hill 2500 Garden Road Monterey, CA 93940	$200.00
Employee Aptitude Survey #9	Educational & Industrial Testing Service Box 7324, San Diego, CA 92107	$16.00
VALPAR 4	VALPAR Corporation 3801 East 34th Street Tucson, AZ 85713	$975.00
VALPAR 8		$1375.00
WEST Bus Bench	Work Evaluation Systems Technology 1950 Freeman Long Beach CA 90804	$575.00
WEST 2 Lifting Evaluation		$1040.00
WEST 4 Torquing Strength		$895.00
WEST Tool Sort		
WEST Tool Sort		$89.00
BTE Work Simulator	Baltimore Therapeutic Equipment Company 1201 Bernard Drive Baltimore MD 21223	$25,000.00 or $550/mo.
JAMAR Dynamometer	Fred Sammons, Inc. Box 32, Brookfield, IL 60513-0032	$200.00
Pinch Gauge		$230.00
Snellen Eye Chart	Can be obtained through any local college of optometry.	

stamina, endurance, work place tolerance, and worker behaviors. The typical length of the EWTS Battery is 1 to 1½ days, and the CWTE from 5 to 10 days. Both approaches use carefully selected standardized evaluation tools that are available in the public domain. These evaluation tools can be classified into three categories and are listed below (See Table 12-1 for information regarding sources of availability and approximate cost).

1. Psychometric tests of motor speed and dexterity

"...are designed to measure ability to rapidly and accurately manipulate tools and objects of various sizes and shapes in order to predict job performance. They are usually statistically standardized by comparison to industrial workers."[1]

The psychometric tests selected for use are the Crawford Small Parts Dexterity Test, Bennett Hand Tool Dexterity Test, Minnesota Rate of Manipulation Test, and the Employee Aptitude Survey #9.

2. Demand structured work samples

"...are standardized, highly structured simulated work tasks involving materials and tools that are similar or identical to those in an actual job or cluster of jobs."[1] The commercially available work samples selected for data collection on a work demand relevant basis are the *VALPAR 4, VALPAR 8,* and *WEST Bus Bench.*

3. Work Capacity Evaluation Devices (WCEDs)

"...are pieces of equipment that simulate specific work demands and which can be structured to present evaluation tasks that gradually increase the physical demands made upon the evaluee."[1]

The selected WCEDs are the *WEST 4 Upper Extremity Torquing Strength, WEST 2 Lifting Evaluation* and the *BTE Work Simulator.* By virtue of its cost, the BTE Work Simulator is an optional item.

In addition, the following equipment are used: the *JAMAR Dynamometer,* the *Pinch Gauge,* the *WEST Tool Sort,* and the *Snellen Eye Chart.*

All standardized assessments are administered according to the procedure specified in the manual for that assessment. However, the tests are administered with the basic assumption that the evaluee's performance is affected by the physical demands of the measurement process. These physical demands may include sitting, standing, repetitive or sustained horizontal reaching, forearm supination/pronation, finger/hand grasp and release, visual motor concentration, and so on. During each test administration, the evaluee's responses to the physical demands presented by the test are carefully observed and monitored.

The CWTE uses all the evaluation tools listed and, in addition, employs structured work simulations. These consist of "...workstations located in the evaluation facility that replicate a cluster of job tasks in a realistic manner. These tasks are presented in a graded manner using the actual tools and materials employed in work settings."[1]

Structured work simulations that have been successfully used include electronics assembly, clerical tasks, light industrial assembly, packaging, industrial sewing, manufacture of leather goods, light woodworking, light sheet metal fabrication, pantograph engraving, drafting, janitorial, cosmetician, quality control, and light to moderately heavy materials handling. An attempt is made to replicate relevant environmental, physical, and social characteristics of each job as realistically as is practical. The evaluee's performance is graded on the basis of industrial standards for quality and quantity of productivity. Some, but not all, of the tasks presented can be commercially available work samples (for example, the VALPAR 16 for drafting and the VALPAR 10 for quality control). The factors observed and monitored during performance of structured work simulations include productivity, work tolerances in response to sustained or repetitive physical demands, workplace tolerance, concentration, instructability, safety, and interpersonal behavior.

The EWTS Battery and CWTE together combine aspects of both the "work tests" and "physical capacities evaluation" approaches. The evaluation findings also can be keyed into the DOT so that they can be used as a reference to aid in job matching.

Appropriate Candidates For Work Tolerance Screening

The methods of work tolerance screening presented in this chapter are generally used with evaluees who have successfully worked in the past, and so had established worker role identity and appropriate worker behaviors at one time. However, due to an acute psychological episode or a work injury, the evaluee became disabled. The work tolerance screening helps to determine if the work role identity, fallen into disuse, is still present and operating, or if the evaluee needs assistance to regain the worker role. The screening generally is less useful for psychiatrically or developmentally disabled adolescents who have never established a worker role. Other assessment models with a developmental basis are more appropriate in these cases.

The brief EWTS Battery is used when there is a reasonable expectation that the evaluee's physical and psychological symptoms are well-controlled and that the individual is ready to participate in a job training program or in competitive employment. If the physical or psychological symptoms are unstable, or the evaluee is severely deconditioned, then a brief evaluation that allows for a limited sample of performance ability will not be sufficient to reliably predict productivity, work place tolerance, safety, interpersonal behavior, and other worker behaviors. In this situation, the CWTE is appropriate because it allows for monitoring of a broader sample of performance over a longer period of time.

The Work Tolerance Screening Sequence

1. Clarify the goals of referral and the questions to be answered by means of the evaluation process.

2. Review the most recent medical reports from all significant practitioners, including physicians and rehabilitation personnel.

3. Through interview, obtain the evaluee's report of present functional status, including present ADL function, basic physical tolerances, and limiting psychological or physical symptoms. Other relevant information is medication used, assistive devices needed, gait, hand dominance, other medical problems, and current vocational goals.

4. Develop an Individual Work Evaluation Plan (IWEP) that lists the specific areas of function to be evaluated, the evaluation goals for each area of function, and the evaluation tools to be used. Specify the individual staff member who will be responsible for conducting each aspect of the evaluation.

5. The signing of a Performance Limits Agreement is recommended. This document simply lists permitted limits for sustained sitting or standing, stair climbing, lifting, bending, or whatever is deemed appropriate. By signing this agreement, the evaluee agrees to exceed these limits only by instruction of staff members. This helps reinforce in the evaluee that playing around with equipment, moving furniture, lifting heavy objects, etc. without staff supervision is not permissible.

6. Orient the evaluee to the evaluation program. Provide a clear explanation of rules, time tables, and responsibilites during the course of the evaluation, including timeliness, regular attendance, notification of absences, proper dress, reporting of symptoms or problems, conduct with other evaluees, and so on.

7. Conduct the evaluation.

8. Following completion of the evaluation, arrange an exit conference to be attended by the evaluee, referrer, and evaluator(s). The results of the evaluation are presented and discused with reference to the referral questions.

9. Write the report.

Administering the ERIC Work Tolerance Screening Battery

Section #1: Functional Limitations

Procedure. Perform gross range of motion testing. The motions most commonly tested are arms over head; arms over head/hands behind head; arms behind back at waist height; flexion/extension of elbows, wrists, and fingers; thumb opposition and abduction; forearm supination/pronation; crouching; kneeling; and bending.

Perform any other gross range of motion, strength, or sensation testing indicated by the presence of a diagnosis indicating neurological or musculoskeletal impairment.

If the evaluee is 50 years old or older, has a diagnosis or suspected diagnosis of high blood pressure, low blood pressure, heart dysfunction, pulmonary dysfunction, or severe deconditioning, perform a brief cardiovascular screening. Record heart rate and blood pressure at rest, during a five minute walk at a normal pace, and post activity. Note particularly the presence of irregular pulse, tachycardia, or hypertension.

Section #2: Visual Acuity

Evaluation Equipment. Snellen Eye Chart

Procedure. Position the evaluee at a distance of 20 feet from the chart, which is mounted on a wall. Evaluate with glasses or contacts if normally worn.

Have the evaluee cover the left eye and, beginning at the top, read the letters on the chart using the right eye. Repeat with the right eye covered, then with both eyes uncovered.

Score the test: the smallest line of letters read denotes the level of visual acuity.

Section #3: Psychophysical Limitations

Equipment. WEST Tool sort

Procedure. Before beginning, read the manual that comes with the test.

Instruct the evaluee to sort each card according to perceived physical ability to use the tool pictured on the card. For this evaluation, the skill required to handle the tool need not be considered.

After the cards have been sorted, debrief the evaluee by selecting representative tools from each category and ask the evaluee to explain his reasoning behind placing each tool in the chosen category. The purpose of the debriefing is to uncover work function themes: those usually unstated rules that each evaluee uses to guide his participation in work activities.

Observations. Indications of an unrealistic perception of ability to use tools. The evaluees may have a self-perception of being more or less physically capable than they really are.

Section #4: Sitting, Horizontal Reaching, Motor Coordination, Fine Dexterity

Equipment. Employee Aptitude Survey #9, Crawford Small Parts Dexterity Test

Procedure. Carefully read the manual that comes with each test.

Position the evaluee in a seated position at a table or desk, facing the test. Ensure that the evaluee can sit with good posture and that lighting is adequate.

Instruct the evaluee according to the task to be performed.

Administer and score the tests as described in the manual(s) and observe and monitor the evaluee's performance.

Observations. Duration of sitting tolerance.

Posture and positioning, including slouching, forward bending, leaning to one side, supporting weight on the upper extremities.

Skill and dexterity for manipulating small parts and tools, prehension patterns, and the presence of intention tremors.

Abnormal posturing of the hand, wrist, elbow, shoulder, or head due to weakness, fatigue, lack of flexibility, or to avoid discomfort.

Behavioral or verbal displays of physical or psychological discomfort, including aching, fatigue, sharp pain, tingling, stiffness, inability to concentrate, frustration.

Cognitive factors, including instructability, attention span, concentration, frustration tolerance.

Section #5: Standing, Horizontal Reaching, Medium Dexterity

Equipment. Bennett Hand Tool Dexterity Test, Minnesota Rate of Manipulation Test VALPAR 4, VALPAR 8, WEST Bus Bench

Procedure. Carefully read the manual that comes with each test.

Position the evaluee in a standing position at a workbench, facing the test. Adjust the work height so that the evaluee can stand with good posture.

Instruct the evaluee according to the task to be performed.

Administer and score the tests as described in the manual(s) and observe and monitor the evaluee's performance.

Observations. Duration of standing tolerance.

Posture and positioning, including slouching, forward bending, leaning to one side, supporting weight on the upper extremities, and standing on one foot.

Skill and dexterity for manipulating medium sized parts and tools, prehension patterns, and the presence of intention tremors.

Abnormal posturing of the hand, wrist, elbow, shoulder, or head due to weakness, fatigue, lack of flexibility, or to avoid discomfort.

Behavioral or verbal displays of physical or psychological discomfort, including aching, fatigue, sharp pain, tingling, stiffness, inability to concentrate, frustration.

Cognitive factors, including instructabilty, attention span, concentration, memory, planning, frustration tolerance, and problem-solving.

Section #6: Strength and Endurance for Resistive Tool Handling

Equipment. JAMAR Dynamometer, Pinch Gauge, WEST 4 Upper Extremity Strength for Torquing, BTE Work Simulator or weighted box and push/pull gauge

Procedure. Carefully read the manual that comes with each piece of equipment.

Position the evaluee in a standing position at a workbench, facing the test. For the JAMAR evaluation, the evaluee faces the evaluator. Adjust the work height so that the evaluee can stand with good posture.

Instruct the evaluee according to the task to be performed.

Administer and score the tests of gripping, pinching, torquing and pushing/pulling with tools as described in the manual(s), and observe and monitor the evaluee's performance, with the following special instructions:

For the JAMAR Dynamometer grip strength test, measure the evaluee's grip strength in three repetitive trials, alternating from the dominant to the non-dominant hand, over each of the five grip settings on the dynamometer. There will be a total of 15 gripping trials for each hand. When this procedure is used, the evaluator can gather data regarding endurance for gripping, consistency of grip effort, and the ideal grip span or handle size for the evaluee. The percentile score[10] is based on the highest grip measurement obtained for each hand.

When measuring finger strength with the Pinch Gauge, both lateral and palmar pinch are measured in three repetitive trials, alternating from the dominant to the non-dominant hand. The percentile score[10] is based on the highest pinch measurments obtained for each hand.

During the WEST 4 Upper Extremity Torquing Strength test, the evaluee uses a standard nutdriver with a 1-in diameter handle while the evaluator turns an adjustment screw to gradually increase the amount of resistance presented to the evaluee. The maximum resistance overcome by the evaluee is then measured in inch-pounds using a torque measuring nutdriver. Three measurements are obtained for the left and right hands for torquing in both supination and pronation, to assess endurance and consistency of effort. The percentile score is based on the highest strength measurement of three trials.

To set up the BTE Work Simulator to measure pushing/pulling strength, turn on the machine and set the controls on the left side of the control panel to read "manual" and "dynamic." On the right side of the control panel, turn the knob that adjusts the exercise level all the way counterclockwise.

Place the "ratchet" switch at the center setting, so that the shaft provides resistance in both directions. Push the "advance" button about seven times, until "set ratchet position" shows on the control panel. Set the shaft in a horizontal position and insert tool #801 (lever) in the shortest position. Position the evaluee so that the BTE shaft is to the evaluee's right. Have the evaluee grasp the vertical handle and alternately push and pull the lever while the resistance is gradually increased using the exercise level knob. Stop at the point that the evaluee has to use the assistance of body weight to move the lever. Measure in pounds the horizontal force exerted. Repeat with the left upper extremity.

Pushing/pulling strength with the upper extremities also can be measured with a rigid box resembling a milk crate with handle slots and covered on the bottom with durable felt or carpet. Place the box on a smooth-surfaced table, and have the evaluee first grasp the box with the right hand and push/pull while the evaluator gradually adds weight to the box. Stop at the point that the evaluee has to use the assistance of body weight to move the box. Measure in pounds the horizontal force exerted. Repeat with the left upper extremity.

Horizontal force can be most accurately measured using a push/pull gauge, available from major industrial supply companies. The JAMAR dynamometer can be used as a push/pull gauge by slowly pressing its inside handle against the lever or box handle until the lever or box moves. Horizontal force in pounds is then read on the JAMAR dial. A spring scale or even a bathroom scale, although less accurate, can be used to measure horizontal force. The spring scale is attached to the lever or box handle and slowly pulled, while the bathroom scale is held against the lever or side of the box and slowly pushed.

Observations. Grasping patterns. Strength and endurance for applying squeezing/gripping, torquing, or pushing/pulling force with tools. Limiting factors may be weakness, muscular or cardio-vascular deconditioning, or pain. Overall strength can be categorized as being below average and suitable for light industrial or clerical work, or average or above average and suitable for industrial work requiring application of moderate or heavy resistance with tools. Determination of strength range for gripping or torquing can be made using the percentile scores. With regard to pushing/pulling force with tools, 5 lbs to 10 lbs generally may be considered in the light range, 15 lbs to 25 lbs in the moderate range, and 30 lbs or greater in the heavy range.

Behavioral or verbal displays of physical discomfort, including muscular or joint pain, fatigue, dizziness, shortness of breath, or chest pain.

Indications of severe deconditioning. Resting pulse and blood pressure, as well as measurement of heart rate and blood pressure response to activity can be used to help make this determination.

Any "danger signs" that might mean that an injured hand, arm, back, knee, or heart is being overstressed. Discontinue the activity when such signs are observed.

Section #7: Whole Body Pushing/Pulling

Equipment. BTE Work Simulator or industrial container and push/pull gauge

Procedure. If using the BTE Work Simulator, set up the equipment as for Section #6, only position the evaluee with both hands on the vertical handle of the lever and instruct him to push and pull to maximum capability, using upper extremity strength and body weight. Increase the resistance until the evaluee can barely move the lever, and measure horizontal force as described in Section #6.

The "industrial container" that can be used in place of the BTE Work Simulator can be a flat industrial cart or a large sled-like construction of wood on runners covered with durable felt or carpet. Place the industrial container on a smooth-surfaced floor, and have the evaluee grasp it with both hands and push while the evaluator gradually adds weight to the container. Stop at the point that the evaluee can barely move the container. Measure the horizontal force exerted as described in Section #6. Repeat with the evaluee pulling the container.

Observations. Grasping patterns.

Strength and endurance for applying whole body pushing and pulling force. Limiting factors may be weakness, muscular or cardiovascular deconditioning or pain. Generally speaking, multiplying the pushing/pulling force by 10 gives the approximate weight that can be pushed on a wheeled industrial cart over a level, smooth floor. For example, a horizontal pushing force of 20 lbs is approximately the force used to push a 200-lb load just described. Approximately 5 lbs to 15 lbs of horizontal force is considered in the light range, 20 lbs to 35 lbs in the moderate range, and 40 lbs and greater in the heavy range.

Behavioral or verbal displays of physical discomfort, including muscular or joint pain, fatigue, dizziness, shortness of breath, or chest pain.

Indications of severe deconditioning. Resting pulse and blood pressure, as well as measurement of heart rate and blood pressure response to activity can be used to help make this determination.

Any "danger signs" that might mean that an injured hand, arm, back, knee, or heart is being overstressed. Discontinue the activity when such signs are observed.

Section #8: Vertical Reaching, Crouching/Kneeling, Stooping

Equipment. WEST 2, Brief Tool Use Evaluation

Procedure. Carefully read the manual that comes with the WEST 2. Select the evaluation called "brief tool use."

Respect and abide by any physician's restrictions with regard to reaching, kneeling, stooping, or bending.

Position the evaluee in a standing position facing the testing equipment. Using the WEST 2 frame, determine the heights from the floor, in inches, of the evaluee's head, shoulders, chest, waist, knuckles, and knees.

Instruct the evaluee according to the task to be performed.

Administer and score the test as described in the manual and observe and monitor the evaluee's performance.

Observations. The heights at which the evaluee is able to work comfortably, especially with regard to his tolerances for reaching above eye level, kneeling, crouching, or stooping.

The body positions used at various work heights.

Prehension patterns, skill, and dexterity for performing manipulation in various arm positions.

Abnormal or off-balance postures/positions due to weakness, fatigue, lack of flexibility, or pain.

Behavioral or verbal displays of discomfort, including aching, fatigue, dizziness, sharp pain, tingling, stiffness.

Body mechanics and posture for various work positions, including unstable or unbalanced positioning.

Indications of severe deconditioning. Resting pulse and blood pressure, as well as measurement of heart rate and blood pressure response to activity can be used to help make this determination.

Any "danger signs" that might mean that an injured hand, arm, back, knee, or heart is being overstressed. Discontinue the activity when such signs are observed.

Section #9: Lifting (Range of Motion Under Load)

Equipment. WEST 2 Range of Motion Under Load

Procedure. Before beginning, carefully read the manual that comes with the testing equipment. This evaluation is a continuation of Step #8.

Respect and abide by any physician's restrictions with regard to lifting.

Instruct the evaluee according to the tasks to be performed.

Administer and the WEST Standard Lifting Evaluation as described in the manual and observe and monitor the evaluee's performance.

Observations. Grasping patterns used to handle each weight level, and tolerance of sustained grasp of the weight.

The heights at which the evaluee is able to comfortably lift and place each gradation of weight.

The body positions used, especially with regard to ability to reach, crouch, kneel, or stoop while handling weight, as well as abnormal or off-balance postures/positions due to weakness, fatigue, lack of flexibility, or pain.

Body mechanics while handling weight, including unstable or unsafe positioning. The evaluee should not be allowed to continue the evaluation if unsafe or unstable body mechanics are observed and cannot or will not be be corrected by the evaluee.

Behavioral or verbal displays of discomfort, including aching, fatigue, dizziness, sharp pain, tingling, stiffness.

Indications of severe deconditioning. Resting pulse and blood pressure, as well as measurement of heart rate and blood pressure response to activity, can be used to help make this determination.

Any "danger signs" that mean an injured hand, arm, back, knee, or heart is being overstressed. Discontinue the activity when such signs are observed.

Section #10: Carrying

Equipment. Box, Toolbox

Procedure. Determine the weight to be carried. Start with about 50% of the maximum weight handled bilaterally as well as unilaterally during testing of lifting, as described in Section #9.

Determine the height from which the weight is to be lifted and carried, based on evaluation of range of motion under load, as described in Section #9. The weight will either be lifted and carried from the floor or from table or bench height.

Starting with the bilateral lift/carry, have the evaluee lift the selected beginning weight from the selected height and carry it for 100 feet, and then set it back down. Increase the weight by 5 lbs and repeat. Increase by 5 lbs and repeat again. As the weight becomes heavier, the evaluee may be unable to carry it a full 100 feet. Have the evaluee set the weight down if he feels too fatigued to carry it further. Record the distance the weight was carried. Stop at the evaluee's maximum weight, as determined by the WEST Standard Evaluation.

Repeat the sequence with a unilateral lift/carry, with the evaluee using the dominant, or strongest, upper extremity.

Observations. Grasping patterns used to handle each weight level, and tolerance of sustained grasp of the weight.

The distances which the evaluee is able to comfortably carry each gradation of weight.

The gait used while carrying weight, as well as abnormal or off-balance gait due to weakness, fatigue, lack of flexibility, or pain.

Body mechanics while handling weight, including unstable or unsafe positioning. The evaluee should not be allowed to continue the evaluation if unsafe or unstable body mechanics are observed and cannot or will not be be corrected by the evaluee.

Behavioral or verbal displays of discomfort, including aching, fatigue, dizziness, sharp pain, tingling, stiffness.

Indications of severe deconditioning. Resting pulse and blood pressure, as well as measurement of heart rate and blood pressure response to activity, can be used to help make this determination.

Any "danger signs" that mean an injured hand, arm, back, knee, or heart is being overstressed. Discontinue the activity when such signs are observed.

Section #11: Walking

Procedure. Accompany the evaluee on a 10 to 15 minute brisk walk outside, or have the evaluee walk a marked course in a building or a patio area while being observed.

Observations. Walking gait and pace.
Duration of walking tolerance.
Behavioral or verbal displays of physical discomfort, including muscular or joint pain, fatigue, dizziness, shortness of breath, or chest pain.
Indications of severe deconditioning. Resting pulse and blood pressure, as well as measurement of heart rate and blood pressure response to activity, can be used to help make this determination.

Section #12: Climbing

Equipment. Stairs, Ladder (optional)

Procedure. Accompany the evaluee while he climbs one flight of stairs. The evaluee may use the handrail and use his most comfortable pace. After a brief pause, have the evaluee climb an additional flight of stairs if the first flight was tolerated well, and then descend the two flights.
If indicated in the evaluation plan, have the evaluee climb and descend a stable, A-frame type of ladder.

Observations. Climbing gait, pace, and tolerance.
Behavioral or verbal displays of physical discomfort, including muscular or joint pain, fatigue, dizziness, shortness of breath, or chest pain.
Any "danger signs" that might mean that an injured hand, arm, back, knee, or heart is being overstressed. Discontinue the activity when such signs are observed.
Indications of severe deconditioning. Resting pulse and blood pressure, as well as measurement of heart rate and blood pressure response to activity, can be used to help make this determination.

Procedure For Administering The Comprehensive Work Tolerance Evaluation

Step #1

Procedure. Select a structured work simulation to be assigned to the evaluee. Choice can be made on the basis of strongest physical tolerance, cognitive, and skill areas, interest level, and goal of referral. The idea is to choose an activity that presents a high probability of successful completion. Upon completion of the initial tasks, assign additional tasks graded as to level of difficulty.

Position the evaluee, standing or sitting, at table or workbench. Ensure that the evaluee can sit with good posture and that lighting is adequate. Instruct the evaluee according to the task or tasks to be performed. Observe and monitor the evaluee's performance.

Observations. Duration of sitting, standing, and sustained activity tolerance. Sustained activity tolerance is defined as time spent being productive, as opposed to time spent taking a break.

Posture and positioning, including slouching, forward bending, leaning to one side, supporting weight on the upper extremities.

Skill and dexterity in manipulating parts and tools.

Behavioral or verbal displays of physical or psychological discomfort, including aching, fatigue, sharp pain, tingling, stiffness, inability to concentrate, frustration.

Cognitive factors, including instructability, attention span, concentration, memory, planning, frustration tolerance, and problem-solving.

Worker traits, including quality and quantity of productivity, attendance, timeliness, work place tolerance, judgment, safety, interpersonal behavior, and attitude.

Step #2

Introduce the ERIC Work Tolerance Screening Battery throughout the course of the evaluation, as tolerated by the evaluee. This method helps to keep endurance problems from being a threat to reliability.

Case Example

Carol W. is a 42-year-old woman who was working as a field supervisior for a manufacturer of testing equipment when she was injured on September 20, 1982. On the date of injury, she was attacked during a robbery at her place of work and violently slammed into cabinets and counters.

Two days following the incident, she was examined by an orthopedist. It was determined that she had suffered post-traumatic head syndrome, musculoligamentous sprain strain of the lumbar and cervical spine, and right knee injury. Physical therapy was prescribed. Several months later, she developed severe migraine headaches. A CAT scan and lumbar myelogram showed that she had a herniated lumbar disc. She continued to complain of neck, left arm, and lower back pain. The herniated lumbar disc was treated with chymopapain injection in February of 1984, which resulted in some improvement in the lower back. She underwent surgical repair of the right knee in September of 1982.

In August of 1985, Ms. W. started to experience "attacks" that began with nausea, followed by anxiety and depression with a sense of hopelessness, then severe migraine-type headaches lasting 24 hours that caused sensitivity to light and blurring of vision. These attacks occurred about twice a week and continued to worsen week by week until they were of such severity that she was unable to take care of herself. No neurological explanation for these attacks could be found. A psychiatric consult was ordered in September of 1985. During the initial interview, Ms. W. described tension, anxiety, depression, and nightmares. Due to the severity of her symptoms, she was admitted for inpatient therapy at a psychiatric hospital. During the course of her treatment, the following story unfolded:

Ms. W. was adopted. Her childhood was marked by poverty as well as abuse and neglect by her mother. She had a very hard life, yet maintained her psychiatric function throughout her childhood and graduated from high school with average grades. Her mother later developed Alzheimer's disease and the client took care of her for 11 years until she died when the client was 33 years old. The client had two bad marriages in which she was abused physically and emotionally. Her third and current marriage was a reasonably supportive one. She has two grown daughters and a son. Ms. W. was fired minutes after the time of injury, but presumably this had been planned for some time, as she had been there only six weeks and the company had been planning to replace her with a more experienced person. This caused the family considerable financial hardship.

According to the psychiatrist, Ms. W. had demonstrated impressive courage and integrity in the midst of painful life episodes. He stated that a life history such as the client's often predisposes an individual to serious post-traumatic stress disorder.

The psychiatrist's diagnosis was post-traumatic stress disorder, chronic, moderate to severe in degree, and narcissistic personality disorder, slightly above light in degree.

Following one month of hospitalization and four months of outpatient therapy, Ms. W. was referred for vocational rehabilitation. Comprehensive vocational testing was performed in April of 1985, including aptitudes and interests. She demonstrated high average reasoning ability, above average verbal skills, average arithmetic skills, and low average clerical skills and spatial reasoning. She needed to frequently change positions during the testing period to control pain. Symptoms reported included cervical pain radiating to the left arm, tingling and numbness of the left hand, low back discomfort, right knee pain, and fatigue. The symptoms increased cumulatively throughout the day. Her overall performance was good despite the symptoms, indicating numerous areas of potential vocational pursuit. However, Ms. W. stated at the time of the evaluation that she had had no idea whether she was physically capable of working. She was therefore referred for Comprehensive Work Tolerance Evaluation on March 3, 1986.

Ms. W. arrived early for the intake interview. She was dressed in fashionable, businesslike clothing that included color-coordinated accessories and attractive makeup and hair style. She was 66 inches tall and weighed 172 lbs, making her somewhat overweight. She indicated that she was able to perform shopping, cooking, laundry, and light housekeeping chores, but needed assistance with tasks requiring stooping, crouching, or reaching overhead, such as heavier cleaning, vacuuming, and changing the bed linen. She stated that her family helped with heavier chores. Ms. W. reported that she walked up to a mile per day for exercise and that she took no medication other than aspirin and vitamins. During the interview, Ms. W. was cheerful and answered questions willingly, but appeared worried over the outcome of the evaluation. Her movements appeared guarded, and she avoided turning her head. Her sitting posture was erect on the edge of the chair. Due to her physical injuries, Ms. W.'s physician recommended that she be limited to semi-sedentary work and should be precluded from repetitive lifting, pushing, or bending as well as prolonged maintenance of posture with the hands raised or with the neck in prolonged extension position.

Ms. W. began her evaluation on March 4 and concluded on March 17, 1986. She attended all 10 scheduled days of her Comprehensive Work Tolerance Evaluation. She left one hour early on March 6 due to a cervical muscle spasm and arrived late on March

13 due to her car breaking down. She developed a dependable work place tolerance of five hours by the first week and gradually increased until she reached a work place tolerance of seven hours by the last three days of her evaluation. Ms. W. was fully cooperative with staff, participated with marked enthusiam in the evaluation process, and was generally believed by staff to have put forth maximum effort to benefit from the evaluation.

Selected work simulation projects were assigned to Ms. W. during the evaluation. She used a computer terminal for data entry, accounting, and word processing tasks, a Xerox copy machine, a two-and three-hole punch, an office stapler, a 10-key adding machine for simple bookkeeping, and a typewriter for general office use. She performed filing, collating, and assembling of folders. Speed of performance was average and quality was above average. She practiced basic supervisory and teaching skills with other clients, demonstrating above average interpersonal and leadership skills. Her abilities to use proper body mechanics, pace herself for symptom control, receive and follow instructions, concentrate on work tasks, accept supervision, respond to constructive criticism, and work independently were all acceptable for competitive employment. Dexterity testing was attempted, but the client could not complete the tests due to symptomatic response to repetitive upper extremity reaching.

Results of Testing

Sustained Activity Tolerance—Ms. W. was able to sustain work activity without a non-scheduled break for 120 minutes on a dependable basis. Her productivity/work pace during this activity was in the competitive employment range. Optimal sustained activity tolerance was achieved with varied self-paced work tasks that could be performed while alternating approximately 15 to 25 minutes of sitting with 10 to 15 minutes of standing.

Sitting—On a recurring basis, Ms. W. was able to sit for 15 to 25 minutes and could return to sitting after two minutes of walking. On a maximum length basis, Ms. W. was able to sit for 45 minutes. Optimal sitting tolerance was achieved at a standard height work surface with an office chair that was designed ergonimically, preferably with padded armrests. Her primary limitation was reported left-leg numbness with "pins and needles" reported in the ball of the foot, and bilateral fatigue and aching in the shoulders and upper back.

Standing—Ms. W. was able to work while standing for 15 mintues on a recurrent basis and could return to standing after 5 to 10 minutes of sitting or walking. On a maximum length basis, she was able to stand for 30 minutes. Her primary limitation was reported heaviness in the ankles, weakness in the legs, and restlessness.

Lifting—A modified form the the WEST lifting evaluation was used to safely assess Ms. W.'s current lifting capacity. In a bilateral frontal lift, she was able to lift books weighing a maximum of 7 lbs from desk to counter height (30 to 42 inches) on an infrequent basis. Her primary limiting factor for increasing load was reported pulling in the back of the neck with left-hand tingling. In terms of maximum range of motion in a bilateral lift, she was able to lift/lower 5 lbs from desk to chest height (30 to 42 inches) on an infrequent basis. Ms. W.'s primary limitation for increasing range was reported neck strain in the higher range and symptomatic response to bending, stooping, or crouching in the lower range. Her potential to improve maximum lifting capacity appeared to be poor.

Carrying—Ms. W. was able to carry books weighing 7 lbs for 100 feet in a bilateral frontal position on an occasional basis. Optimal bilateral carry was 5 lbs for 100 feet on an occasional basis. Her primary limitation was reported neck pain and left-hand tingling.

Climbing—Ms. W. was able to climb one flight of stairs on an occasional basis at a slow pace while using the handrail.

Stooping/Kneeling/Crouching—Ms. W. had difficulty bending to reach below waist level due to symptomatic response to activity. She could not crouch due to the previous knee injury. She refused to attempt to kneel. Ms. W. was able to stoop slowly, with reported pain, while holding on to a stable object for balance and support, to retrieve an object from below knee height. She needed an assistive device, or a chair or stool, to retrieve light objects from the floor or reach into lower drawers or shelves.

Reaching—Ms. W. was able to reach vertically to shoulder height (54 inches) on an occasional basis, and to eye level on a brief intermittent basis, limited by reported neck pain. In horizontal reaching tasks, she was able to reach across a work surface beyond 12 inches from her body on an occasional basis. She needed her forearms supported while working whenever possible. Her primary limitation was reported neck and bilateral shoulder pain.

Handling—Ms. W. was able to perform tasks characteristic of an office setting as follows:

1. Collating and stapling—Ms. W. assembled and stapled 60 packets and could resume the task after doing an alternate task for 60 minutes. Limiting factor was reported cervical and left-hand pain.

2. Sorting papers, hole punching, and inserting in a binder—Ms. W. was able to perform this task continuously for 60 minutes, limited by reported cervical and left-hand pain.

3. Typing an a computer keyboard—Tolerance was 15 to 30 minutes, limited by reported cervical and left-hand pain.

4. Ten-key calculator with the right hand—Ms. W.'s tolerance was 30 minutes, limited by reported cervical pain.

5. Filing—Ms. W. was able to file for 10 minutes continuously, and sat on a stool to help her reach the lower drawers.

6. Continuous writing—Ms. W.'s tolerance was 15 minutes, limited by reported cervical pain. She benefited from having a slanted surface to write on in order to avoid neck flexion.

Although Ms. W. had special needs with regard to the physical demands of work that she was able to tolerate, it was concluded that she was potentially employable on the basis of the quality of her work, her interpersonal and supervisiory skills, and her other aptitudes. Based on the findings of the Comprehensive Work Tolerance Evaluation, it was recommended that Ms. W. would be able to achieve work place tolerance and productivity acceptable for employment with varied, self-paced office tasks combined with supervisory duties.

Conclusions and Recommendations

The case just presented is an example of an industrial rehabilitation client with a secondary psychiatric diagnosis. It is the author's experience that many adult psychiatric patients need assistance to return to the worker role. Some are housewives recently divorced who have not worked since they were teenagers. Some are severely deconditioned, having spent weeks or months in a state of inactivity due to depression. Some have physically handicapping conditions such as lower back or cervical injury, knee injury, diabetes, pulmonary disease, and heart disease. Most are simply unsure of their current emotional and physical capabilites in a work setting.

In the present system, the industrial rehabilitation population is favored in terms of funding for vocational rehabilitation. These clients' cases are managed by rehabilitation nurses and vocational counselors in the private sector. Under the industrial rehabilitation system, management of the medical rehabilitation "patient" and the vocational rehabilitation "client" takes place in one reimbursement system, making transition fairly smooth. Psychiatric patients are usually referred to the state department of rehabilitation for vocational services. The delays and paperwork required to transfer from one reimbursement system to another can be frustrating to the patient and can create financial hardship. Additional delays may occur because counselors often carry heavy caseloads. When a patient is not physically and emotionally ready for vocational rehabilitation, or when the vocational counselor lacks sufficient information on physical capacity and worker traits to make appropriate placement, the patient may then become a "dropout" from vocational rehabilitation. The ultimate result is more delay and considerable financial loss all around.

Summary

Occupational therapists can be of enormous value in the transition from adult psychiatric treatment to vocational rehabilitation, both by helping to determine when a patient is ready to enter vocational rehabilitation, and by supplying information to the vocational counselor. Work tolerance screening can be an important component of a total vocational readiness program for adult psychiatric patients. The current occupational therapy literature is rich regarding work readiness programs for adolescents. Less has been written concerning the vocational readiness needs of adults undergoing psychiatric treatment and the effectiveness of occupational therapy intervention to ease the transition to return to work. Research in this area is much needed, and this is a fertile area for study and program development.

References

1. Matheson LN and Ogden-Niemeyer L (1987). Work Capacity Evaluation. Anaheim, California: Employment and Rehabilitation Institute of California, pp 1-6, VI-1 through VI-37.
2. Stevens AL (1950). Work evaluation in rehabilitation. Occupational Therapy and Rehabilitation 29(3), 157-161.
3. Rosenberg R and Wellerson T (1960). A structured pre-vocational program. Am J Occup Ther 14, 57-60, 106.
4. Pruitt WA (1977). Vocational Evaluation. Menomonie, Wisconsin: Walt Pruitt and Associates.
5. Wegg L (1960). The essentials of work evaluation. Am J Occup Ther 14, 65-69, 79.
6. Reuss EE, Rawe DE, and Sundquist AE (1958). Development of a physical capacities evaluation. Am J Occup Ther 12, 1-14.
7. U.S. Department of Labor (1977). Dictionary of Occupational Titles (Volume 4). Washington D.C.: Superintendent of Documents, U.S. Government Printing Office.

8. Ogden LD and Wright MC (1985). Work-related programs in occupational therapy: A renaissance. The Roles of Occupational Therapy in Continuity of Care. New York: Haworth Press.

9. Harvey-Krefting L (1985). The concept of work in occupational therapy: A historical review. Am J Occup Ther 39, 301-313.

10. Mathiowetz V, Kashman N, Volland G, Weber K, Dowe M, and Rogers S (1985). Grip and pinch strength: Normative data for adults. Archives of Physical Medicine and Rehabilitation 66, 69-74.

CHAPTER 13

RESEARCH ANALYSIS OF OCCUPATIONAL THERAPY ASSESSMENTS USED IN MENTAL HEALTH

Franklin Stein, PhD, OTR, FAOTA

In theory, most clinicians accept the principle that patient evaluation is an integral part of the treatment process in which the occupational therapist plans an individual treatment program based on the results of formal testing and informal interviews.[1] However, in practice, patient evaluation is not used consistently. There is a wide range in the types of evaluations used and the quality of the test instruments in terms of reliability, validity, and standardized scoring. Occupational therapists should use test instruments with regard to standardization procedures, along with the skills necessary to administer and interpret test results. Sometimes custommade tests are needlessly developed by occupational therapists who may not be aware of the existence of already published standardized tests.

The objective of this chapter is to present a cross-section of tests that have been developed by occupational therapists for clinical practice in psychosocial dysfunction. The tests are analyzed from the perspective of a researcher who is concerned with the quantitative issues in measurement and the validity of using those tests with psychiatric populations.

For the occupational therapist, patient evaluation should be a systematic process of measuring function or behavior. It is an integral part of the treatment process in treating the mentally ill client.

Characteristics of a Good Test

The accuracy and precision in evaluating a client's performance or improvement depends upon the quality of the test instrument. What are the characteristics of a good test instrument? Does the test answer the following questions?

1. What is the population for whom the test is targeted (e.g., autistic children, schizophrenic inpatients, drug-dependent clients, or a general psychiatric group)?

2. What are the specific purposes of the test (e.g., planning treatment goals, determining prognosis, establishing baseline data, or documenting progress)?

3. What are the areas of function identified in the test, (e.g., social interactions, prevocational, developmental, leisure interests, perceptual-motor abilities or ADL skills)?

4. What are the methods used to evaluate a patient? Primary sources for evaluating a client include medical records, clinical

observation of patient performance, interview, objective tests, checklists of interests, ADL scales, self-reports, and biomechanical or physiological measurement of human factors.

5. Is there a standardized procedure or manual of instructions in administering the test and interpreting results?

6. Are there special skills or certification that are necessary to administer, score, and interpret results of the test?

7. Is the scale of measurement used in collecting data identifiable (i.e., nominal, ordinal, interval, or ratio)?

8. Are negative factors controlled that can potentially interfere with obtaining reliable test results, such as subject fatigue, anxiety, lack of motivation, acute psychotic symptoms, poor environment for testing, and inadequate intelligence for understanding test instructions?

9. Are research data reported (such as those that are derived from objective studies of the test) including reliability, validity, and normative scores?

Differential Role of Occupational Therapy in Evaluation

Sundberg[2] defined personality assessment "as the set of processes used by a person or persons for developing impressions and images, making decisions and checking hypotheses about another person's pattern of characteristics which determines one's behavior in interaction with the environment."

In general, the major goals of assessment for the occupational therapist include assessment for decision-making in planning a treatment program, and the documentation of improvement, change, or status in the client's behavior. In addition, Cynkin[3] proposed that occupational therapy assessment is designed to establish client needs and to decide whether occupational therapy can help meet these needs.

Although assessment is used by many mental health professionals, such as the psychiatrist, psychologist, social worker, nurse, rehabilitation counselor, and occupational therapist, the methods, content and overall purposes vary. In Table 13-1, the major differences in assessment are compared and specific examples are used to differentiate purposes. In practice much overlap and duplication occurs in the assessment of a client. All mental health professionals are concerned with understanding the client's development, behavior and interaction with family members in the

Table 13-1
Examples of Differential Roles of Mental Health Professionals in Assessment

Profession	Methods Used Usually	Content	Purpose	Examples of Specific Instruments
Psychologist	Paper and pencil objective or projective tests	Personality, performance, intelligence, aptitude, etc,	Dynamic interpretation of human characteristics	—Minnesota Multiphasic Personality Inventory (MMPI) —Thematic Apperception test (TAT) —Stanford-Binet Intelligence Test
Psychiatrist	Psychiatric Interview	Abnormal behavior	Diagnostic	—Diagnostic and Statistical Manual (DSM-III) Criteria for diagnosis
Social Worker	Family interview	Family dynamics	Social-interaction analysis	—Roe-Siegelman Parent-Child Relations Questionnaire
Rehabilitation Counselor	Simulated work tasks	Vocational	Work adjustment	—McCarron-Dial Work Evaluation System
Nurse	Clinical Observation	Ward interaction	Documentation	—Nurse's Observation Scale for Inpatient Evaluation
Occupational Therapist	Activity Tasks	Life skills and competencies	Implementing treatment	—Kohlman Evaluation of Living Skills (KELS) —Bay Area Functional Performance Evaluation (BaFPE)

community. However, because of the nature of the professions and educational preparations, evaluation purposes differ.

Assumptions in Clinical Evaluation

What are some of the assumptions in clinical evaluation that guide a clinician in assessment?

1. Evaluation is an essential factor in the treatment process. It is used to determine the client's abilities, interests, potentials, and work traits.

2. Evaluation is used to establish baseline data.

3. Evaluation is based on reliable and valid instrumentation. The degree of accuracy in measurement is dependent upon the degree of reliability (consistency) and validity (truth).

4. Error is always present to a degree in evaluation due to tester, client, instrument, and environmental factors. Therefore, test data usually approximate the variables that one is testing.

5. The validity of evaluation is increased by eliminating internal and external factors that include client fatigue, lack of motivation, anxiety, and inadequate test setting.

6. Evaluation can provide data for documentation and the basis for establishing efficacy and quality assurance. Evaluation is an excellent method for objectively determining client progress.

Criterion-Referenced Versus Norm-Referenced Tests

In testing circles during the last 20 years there was a growing interest in devising criterion-referenced tests in lieu of norm-referenced tests. Criterion-referenced tests first proposed by Glaser,[4] use content domains for setting standards of performance. For example, if one were going to devise a new test for independent living skills, one would seek to define competence in independent living skills by collecting data from a target population. By collecting data, competence or mastery of independent living skills would be operationally defined. Standards would be established based on these data, and a cut-off point for degree of independence would be statistically fixed. In comparison, in a norm-referenced test, a raw score that an individual obtains on a test is compared to a normative sample. The scores of the normative sample are distributed along a normal curve. In this way, a raw score can be converted into percentile ranks or standard scores.

Table 13-2
Criterion-Referenced vs. Norm-Referenced Test

—absolute standards of competence or mastery are established based on theory	—relative standards are based on normal samples
—scores are derived from standards or behaviors or competency	—scores are compared to established norms
—scores are interpreted, based on what the client can or cannot do and then used diagnotically	—scores are interpreted by percentile ranks, standard scores and organized along a normal curve
—content of items are comprehensive of domain	—content of items are a sample of domain
—cut-off score for passing is based on minimal standards of competency	—cut-off score for passing is based on pre-established percentile rank
—theoretically all can pass or all can fail	—the number of failures is predicted before test is administered

Criterion-referenced tests are based on a comprehensive theory that generates ideas for a specific content domain. In criterion-referenced tests, items are selected systematically to represent the content domain. For example, if an investigator is interested in devising a test of visual perception, the first task is to determine the dimensions of the concept from the theoretical and experiential perspectives. The investigator would use the theoretical framework to guide the writing of test items and afterwards use a representative sample from a target population to define normal visual perception. Operational performance standards are used in writing test items, such as copying a geometrical design or identifying a hidden figure. On the other hand, in devising a norm-referenced test, the investigator selects random items and afterwards collects data from a representative sample. The norm-referenced data can be later organized into age and sex categories.

In summary, a criterion-referenced test is one that is deliberately constructed to yield measurements that are directly interpreted in terms of specific performance standards.[4] On the other hand, norm-referenced tests are "generally employed ...to assess degree of attainment. Some published tests are so constructed to permit both norm-referenced and criterion-referenced applications"[5] (p. 98). A summary of the differences between criterion and norm-referenced tests is given in Table 13-2.

Applying Criterion-Referenced Concepts to Occupational Therapy

The major content areas for occupational therapists in evaluation include for example, basic living skills,[6-9] interests,[10] occupational role,[11] and work behavior.[12] If one uses a criterion-referenced approach to these areas, one should consider the following factors:

1. The theory underlying these concepts is identified.

2. Research evidence supporting any assumptions of the test are stated.

3. The content domain of the test that considers a comprehensive view of skills, interests, and behavior is discussed.

4. The specific target population is operationally defined in terms of age, intelligence, education, and degree of disability.

5. The test items are generated by selecting representative samples of behavior.

6. Performance standards in the test are based on systematically collected data from representative samples of the target population.

7. Test items are pilot-tested for clarity and ease of administration.

8. Scoring methods are devised that are operationally defined.

9. Reliability and validity data are objectively obtained.

10. A test manual for administering, scoring, and interpreting data is provided.

11. The degree of competency in administering the test is included in test description.

Current Survey of Psychosocial Tests for Occupational Therapists

Assessment instruments available to the psychiatric occupational therapist prior to 1970 were usually informal and non-standardized. However, in the last 17 years, major tests were developed by occupational therapists targeted for psychiatric populations. These assessment instruments are changing the practice of psychiatric occupational therapy to a more data based profession. This trend toward the development of standardized tests with reliability and validity data available represents progress in psychiatric occupational therapy practice. Table 13-3 is a summary of test instruments developed specifically for the psychiatric occupational therapist. It is not meant to be a comprehensive survey of all the tests available, but a sample of representative instruments in psychiatric occupational therapy.

Table 13-3
Sample of Psychiatric Occupational Therapy Test Instruments (1962-1987)

Name of Test	Authors	Date Published	Target Population	Major Variables Assessed	Comments
Minnesota Follow-Up Study Rehabilitation Scale	Wolff, R.J.	1961	Adult Psychiatric Patients	Post-discharge Adjustment	Therapist bases judgment on patient observation
Diagnostic Occupational Therapy Test Battery	Andros, L.R. Dreyfus, E.A. Bloesch, M.	1965	Adult Psychiatric Patients	Psychodymanics of Personality	Projective test
Occupational Therapy Trait Rating Scale	Clark, J.R. Koch, R.A. Nichols, R.C.	1965	Adult Psychiatric In-Patients	Behavioral Strengths	Used by therapists to observe patient
Pre-Vocational Evaluation of Rehabilitation Potential	Ethridge, D.A.	1968	Adult Psychiatric In-Patients	Pre-Vocational Abilities	Observation of patient assignments in hospital work assignments
Comprehensive Occupational Therapy Evaluation Scale	Brayman, S.J. Kirby, T. Misenheimer, A.M. Short, M.S.	1968	Adolescent and Adult Psychiatric In-Patients	Behavior while engaging in activity	Observation tool
Comprehensive Evaluation of Basic Living Skills	Casanova, J. Ferber, J.	1976	Chronic Adult Psychiatric In-Patients	Self-Care and Basic Living Skills	Observation tool
Parachek Geriatric Rating Scale	Parachek, J.F. King, L.J.	1976	Geriatric In-Patients	Physical capabilities, Self-care, Social Behavior	Observation tool
Magazine Picture Collage	Lerner, C. Ross, G.	1977	Adult Psychiatric In-Patients	Personality, Ego Functions	Projective test
SBC Adult Psychiatric Sensory Integration Evaluation	Schroeder, C.V. Block, M.P. Trottier, E.C. Stowell, M.S.	1978	Adult Psychiatric In-Patients	Sensory and Motor responses	Based on Jean Ayres' theory of sensory integration

Table 13-3 (continued)
Sample of Psychiatric Occupational Therapy Test Instruments (1962-1987)

Name of Test	Authors	Date Published	Target Population	Major Variables Assessed	Comments
Kohlman Evaluation of Living Skills	Kohlman, L.	1979	Acute Psychiatric In-Patients	Self-care, Living Skills, Work, Leisure	Client is evaluated through task or interview
Bay Area Functional Performance Evaluation	Bloomer, J.S. Williams, S.K.	1979	Adult Psychiatric In-Patients	Functional Abilities and Social Interactions	Self-report is used in collecting data
Independent Living Skills Evaluation	Johnson, T.P. Vinnicombe, B.J. Merril, G.W.	1980	Adult Chronic Psychiatric Out-Patients	Functional Living Skills	Client rates self on skills
B.H. Battery	Hemphill, B.J.	1982	Adult Psychiatric In-Patients	Personality Characteristics	Projective test
Occupational Role History: A Screening Tool for Psychiatric Occupational Therapy	Florey, L.L. Michelman, S.M.	1982	Adult Psychiatric In-Patient	Occupational Role and Leisure Activities	Open ended questionnaire
Maguire's Trilevel* ADL Assessment	Maguire, G.H.	1985	Geriatric	Activities of Daily Living in Person, Home and Community	Interactive scale examining function in client's environment
Assessment of Occupational Functioning*	Watts, J.H. et al.	1986	Geriatric	Values, interests, roles, habits, skills and motivation	
Milwaukee Evaluation of Daily Living Skills*	Leonardelli, C.A.	1987	Adult Chronic Psychiatric	Basic living skills, safety, communication and transportation	Client is evaluated while performing task
Barth Time Construction*	Barth, T.	1987	Adolescent and Adult Psychiatric	Time analyzed in ADL, Work, Leisure and Sleep	Client completes time chart within activity project
The Role Checklist*	Barris, R. Oakley, F. Kielhofner, G.	1987	Adolescents, adults and elderly with physical or psychosocial dysfuntion	Ten major roles in life such as student, worker . . .	Client self-report
NPI Interest* Check List	Rogers, J.C.	1987	Adult Psychiatric In-Patients	Eighty interest items are rated	Client self-report

Outline for Analyzing Tests

The assessments reviewed for this chapter are the following:

A. Minnesota Follow-up Study Rehabilitation Rating Scale (MFS)
B. Diagnostic Occupational Therapy Test Battery
C. Occupational Therapy Trait Rating Scale (OTTRS)
D. Pre-vocational Evaluation of Rehabilitation Potential
E. Comprehensive Evaluation of Basic Living Skills
F. The Independent Living Skills Evaluation ILSE)

These tests were examined from the viewpoint of a researcher in hopes of generating research and stimulating interest in furthering the development of occupational therapy assessments in mental health.

Outline for Reviewing Tests

1. Title:
2. Date Published:
3. Authors:
4. Publisher: Distributor of test or where available
5. Target Population: What was the original sample that data were collected from in terms of age, diagnostic group, and geographical location? Is there a specific target population for which the test is appropriate?
6. Variables Assessed: What are the specific areas of function, behavior, or personality that are being assessed? What are the major stated purposes of the test?
7. Measurement Scales: What is the level of measurement in the test?

   A. Qualitative (subjective judgment)
   i Nominal scale of measurement refers to evaluating variables using independent categories such as can or cannot perform a specific task.
   ii Ordinal scale of measurement refers to evaluating variables using magnitude and ranking such as completely dependent in task, needs assistance, or independent functioning. Variables also can be rated on a numerical scale from 1 to 5, for example, where 1 indicates no self-care and 5 indicates care for self independently.

   B. Quantitative (objective evaluation)
   i Interval scale of measurement refers to scoring variables on a continuous scale with equal distances between score values. Pulse rate, blood pressure, height, and weight are usually measured on interval scales using tests that produce mathematical data.

    ii Ratio scale of measurement incorporates the concept of an absolute zero. Most assessments in psychiatry are qualitative measurements—either nominal scales, such as diagnostic categories, or ordinal scales, such as behavioral rating scales (See Table 13-4).

8. Administration of Instrument: When does the occupational therapist administer the test, such as while the patient is working in the occupational therapy clinic, after observing patient over a specified period of time, or in a separate interview? How long does the test take to administer? Is there special training to administer the test? Are special materials or environments required?

9. Scoring and Interpretation of Results: Is there an overall score or subtest scores derived from the test results? Are there norms available to interpret raw scores? How are the results used in treatment planning, documentation of progress, and discharge recommendations?

10. Test Reliability and Validity: If one assumes that a specific characteristic of an individual remains constant, then a reliable measuring instrument should reflect the stable characteristic over periods of time and through repeated trials.

    Improving the quality of measurement is accomplished by reducing the potential error factors related to the test. Instruments such as the goniometer, electromyelograph, and dynamometer are usually reliable indicators of bodily functions. On the other hand, questionnaires, surveys, rating scales, attitude inventories, and interest tests have comparatively less reliability. By the very nature of the test, the reliability index is affected. Many mechanical instruments that record bodily functions need only be calibrated to be reliable. By comparison, individuals confronted with ambiguous questions, who are inattentive and lacking motivation, will affect reliability.

    In devising a reliable instrument, the investigator must be sensitive to factors in the test, subject taking the test, and the directions in administering the test. All three factors can affect test reliability. Reliability is not a simple concept that merely reflects the accuracy of the instrument. In any test administered to subjects, individual differences such as level of reading ability, need to conform, desire to please the examiner, and anxiety are important factors that will increase the error variance and decrease the consistency of response. Since human beings constantly react to internal and external

Table 13-4
Classification of Scales of Measurement[1]

Measurement Scale	Type of Variable	Item Task	Assumptions	Examples
Nominal	Discrete	Sorting of items into categories	Items are mutually exclusive	Diagnostic and Statistical Manual (DSM-III). Categorizes individuals into diagnostic areas
Ordinal	Discrete	Rank ordering items from high to low	Items are hierarchical in series	Occupational Therapy Trait Rating Scale, 1965. Patients performance during therapy is scored 1 to 5
Interval	Continuous	Selecting test values along a continuum	Threre are equal intervals between raw scores	Stanford-Binet Intelligence Scales. Test assumes results are normally distributed along a continuum.
Ratio	Continuous	Establishing absolute zero point in a continuum	The absolute zero point represents the absence of function in the test scale	Jamar Dynamometer Grip Strength Test. Test scores are continuous with a zero representing lack of grip strength.

[1]Adapted from S.S. Stevens, (1946) Theories of scales of measurement, *Science*, 103, 677-680.

factors, reliability must be interpreted in a relative degree when considering personality tests, questionnaires, and attitude scales. Most researchers with human subjects regard a reliability coefficient of approximately .80 or above as an acceptable level of a test's consistency in measuring a variable.

There are three main techniques for measuring test reliability. In split-half reliability, the test is broken into two equivalent parts, and the sections are correlated with each other. In test-retest reliability, a test is given twice within a specified period of time and the scores on the two tests are correlated. In alternate form reliability, two editions of the same test are compared. The test results are compared for temporal stability and consistency of response.[5]

Another method used is interrater reliability. The results of this method examine both the reliability of the test and the reliability of different test administrators. In this method, the degree of error in the test and the individuals administering the test are evaluated.

Item Analysis—A researcher, in devising a test or in assessing patients, is interested in the effectiveness of individual test items. Those items which are ambiguous and have a low discriminative value are eliminated. Item analysis is a method of gauging the quality of each item. In item analysis, the percentage of passes and failures are calculated for each item.

Another method of anlayzing items is to determine which items had a high correlation to the overall score. This analysis will enable the researcher to separate high and low discriminative value items. This may be particularly important in achievement and aptitude tests.

Test Validity—Validity reflects the authenticity of a test. Does the test measure what it purports to measure? A test may measure a concept consistently, but it may not, in fact, measure what the researcher identifies as the intent of the test. Tests purporting to measure general intelligence, self-image, occupational interests, and attitude toward the disabled actually may be measuring other concepts.

The degree to which a test is valid is the degree of empirical evidence that corroborate the results of a test. Tests or instruments which collect primary data, such as an EMG, x-ray, goniometer, and muscle strength, are easily verified and corroborated. However, tests which collect secondary data, such as personality characteristics derived from multiple factors in the individual, are difficult to validate. Personality, attitude, abilities, and interests are complex variables derived from many facets of the individual's life related to genetics, social learning, cultural identification, and physiological factors.

The researcher seeking to validate a personality test is limited by the ability to corroborate the researcher's findings. Traditionally, validity is established on the following bases:

A. Content validity is the degree to which the test appears to measure a concept by a logical analysis of the items.

B. Concurrent validity is the degree of correlation with another standardized instrument. A new test may be designed because it is less time consuming and less expensive than another established validated instrument.

C. Predictive validity is the degree to which a test can predict success or accuracy over a period of time (longitudinally). A test devised to predict success in a rehabilitation program for stroke patients is an example of predictive validity. In this example, follow-up data from longitudinal studies would determine the correlation between the initial test predictor score and subsequent success in a program.

D. Construct validity is considered to be the highest form of empirical evidence that is most sought by scientific researchers. Construct validity assumes a theoretical rationale underlying the test instrument. In testing an instrument for construct validity, the researcher seeks behavioral data to substantiate the position that the test is in fact measuring a defined variable. For example, an investigator devising a test to measure self-image, would design or apply a theory that underlies the concept. The theory would include developmental factors, relationships with other variables, and predictive behavior. Construct validity is obtained by collecting research data over a period of time. The usefulness of a test in measuring variables such as occupational interests, cognitive skills, and personality, is in its ability to detect changes in the individual.

11. Other Comments: Included in this section are miscellaneous comments such as the theoretical orientation or conceptual framework of the test and its appropriateness for the occupational therapist.

12. References: Includes books, journals, test manuals and other sources where the test has been published or critically evaluated.

Tests to be Analyzed

A. 1. MINNESOTA FOLLOW-UP STUDY REHABILITATION RATING SCALE (MFS)

2. Date Published: 1961
3. Author: Robert J. Wolff, PhD
4. Citation: Wolff, R.J. (1961) A behavior rating scale. AJOT, 15, 13-16
5. Target Population: The instrument was designed to evaluate the effectiveness of pre-discharge and follow-up planning on the post-hospital adjustment of psychiatric clients.
6. Variables Assessed: Three major categories are analyzed in the test, i.e., response to work, activity, or task; response to people; and ability of the patient to care for daily living needs.
7. Measurement Scales: The rater scores the patient on 15 subcategories of the test using a 5-point ordinal scale.
8. Administration of Instrument: The scale is listed in Appendixes G and H.
9. Scoring and Interpretation of Results: The results of the scale are used to evaluate the patient's post-hospital adjustment. The author also indicates that the scale can be used as a prognostic tool to predict successful adjustment.
10. Reliability and Validity Data: Eight trained psychiatric rehabilitation professionals (including occupational therapists) observed and rated 41 psychiatric patients at Fergus Falls State Hospital in Minnesota. Each patient was rated by two individuals. There was an agreement of 89.3% between raters.

    Concurrent validity between the MFS Rehabilitation Rating Scale and the judgment of rehabilitation personnel were tested. A rank order correlation (rho) of .803 was obtained between the total score on the MFS and a 2-point scale of doing "well" or doing "poorly."
11. Other Comments: The author concluded that "The MFS Rehabilitation Rating Scale provides an easy-to-use, fairly objective and reliable method of recording the observed behavior of patients in a rehabilitation therapies setting" (p. 13).

    The MFS Rehabilitation Rating Scale was used retrospectively in a study to evaluate psychiatric client's performance in a Day Treatment Center (Solberg and Chueh, 1976). The result of the study agreed with a prediction that successful performance in occupational therapy in the Day Treatment Center as measured by the MFS Rehabilitation Rating Scale would be significantly related to successful client outcomes, such as holds a volunteer job, attends college, enrolled in specialized vocational training program or is working, at least part time.

12. Reference: Solberg, N. and Chueh, W. (1976) Performance in occupational therapy as a predictor of successful prevocational training. AJOT, 30, 481-186.

B. 1. DIAGNOSTIC OCCUPATIONAL THERAPY TEST BATTERY

2. Date Published: 1965
3. Authors: Le Roy Androes, MD, Edward A. Dreyfus, PhD, and Marianne Bloesch, OTR
4. Citation: Androes, L.R., Dreyfus, E.A. & Bloesch, M. (1965) Diagnostic test battery for occupational therapy. AJOT, 19, 53-59.
5. Target Population: This projective battery incorporating the House-Tree-Person test with ceramics, painting, leather, and woodwork into a diagnostic instrument is intended for psychiatric patients. The test battery was developed at the Topeka VA Hospital in Kansas.
6. Variables Assessed: The authors discuss the potential information that can be derived from each of the six modalities. For example:

   drawing—can provide a measure of compulsivity, maturity, creativity, and spontaneity.

   ceramics—"Patients, both children and adults, express a great many of their psychic conflicts through this modality, such as impulsivity, regressivity, aggresivity, and passivity."

   painting—"...reveals various levels of development, both cognitively and emotionally." The authors also identify conscious and unconscious feelings that are elicited by the patient's free painting.

   leatherwork—fine and gross motor abilities, degree of compulsivity in organizing patterns, concreteness in following directions, and aggressiveness in using tests and pounding the leather.

   woodwork—gross motor skills, ability to follow directions, cognitive processes and planning ability in carrying out task.

7. Measurement Scales: This is a projective test that elicits personality characteristics and emotional responses while the patient engages in activities. The test is unstructured and its effectiveness in revealing the patient's personality dynamics is dependent upon the therapist's skill in observation and insight into the meaning of the patient's responses. Nominal scale data are recorded by the therapist.

8. Administration of Instrument: The test protocol is listed in Appendix I. The authors recommend that the occupational therapist administer the test battery over a two-to four-hour period, divided into two days. The occupational therapist records verbatim all comments made by the patient. Behavioral observations and general impressions are recorded before, during, and after administration of the test battery.

9. Scoring and Interpretation of Results: The authors recommend that the results of the test battery be incorporated into a report that is divided into the following three sections:
   a. Observations—This section includes the patient's appearance, attitude toward the therapist, and attitude toward the tests.
   b. Test Findings—In this section the occupational therapist records the test results describing specific examples of behavior that exemplify personality characteristics.
   c. Occupational Therapy Recommendations—The occupational therapist recommends the therapeutic modalities that are based, indicated on the psychlogical needs of the patient, the interest shown on specific activities, and the goals of treatment.

10. Reliability and Validity Data: Not reported.

11. Other Comments: Although the scoring and interpretation of results are subjective and based upon the degree of clinical insight of the occupational therapist, the test battery can be useful in obtaining information regarding the psychodynamics underlying the patient's behavior. The main purpose of the test battery is to aid the occupational therapist in planning a therapeutic activity program.

12. Reference: Buck, J. (1948) The House-Tree-Person Test. Journal of Clinical Psychology, 4, 151-159.

C. 1. OCCUPATIONAL THERAPY TRAIT RATING SCALE (OTTRS)
2. Date Published: 1965

3. Authors: John R. Clark. PhD, Barbara A. Koch, OTR, and Robert C. Nichols, PhD

4. Citation: Clark. J., Koch. B.A. & Nichols, R.C. (1965) A factor analytically derived scale for rating psychiatric patients in occupational therapy. AJOT, 19, 14-18.

5. Target Population: The scale was developed from an inpatient psychiatric sample of 39 males and 61 females who had a wide range of diagnoses. The majority of the sample were acutely ill and had good prognoses for recovery.

6. Variables Assessed: The main purpose of the scale is to provide valid observations of patients while they engage in activities during occupational therapy. Five broad areas are assessed: creativity; dominance-manipulativeness (in relating to personnel and patients); energy (work output, enthusiasm, and speed); social isolation; and orderliness.

7. Measurement Scale: This is an ordinal scale that uses descriptor terms under numerical categories.

8. Administration of Instrument: The authors recommend that the occupational therapist only rate "those patients whom you know well." It is implied the therapist would use the scale after working with a patient for an unspecified period of time (Appendices J and K).

9. Scoring and Interpretation of Results: The total raw score is obtained from the numerical ratings on the 21 items. The authors suggest possible applications of the results:
   a. As a comprehensive record of the patient's behavior in occupational therapy.
   b. As documentation of progress at different stages of hospitalization.
   c. For diagnostic purposes and treatment planning.
   d. As descriptive research obtaining data that characterize personality variables and various diagnostic categories in relation to five identified factors.

10. Reliability and Validity Data: A concurrent validity study of the rating scale was completed by Lewinsohn and Clark (1965). The following tests were correlated with the Occupational Therapy Trait Rating Scale: Multidimensional Scale for Rating Psychiatric Patients, Interpersonal Checklist, Hospital Adjustment Scale, Minnesota Multiphasic Personality Inventory, IPAT Anxiety Questionnaire, Rotter Incomplete Sentence Blank, Gorham Proverbs Test, Shipley Hartford Retreat Scale, and Figure Drawings.

A Pearson product-moment correlation coefficients , werederived from instruments. The authors conclude that: "The findings provide excellent support for the concurrent validity of three of the factors (creativity, manipulativeness, and social isolation), partial support for one factor (orderliness), and no support for another factor (energy)."

11. Other Comments: The authors implied that they measured the behavioral strengths of the patients that may occur as a function of occupational therapy. They also suggested that the OTTRS measured behavioral characteristics of the patient rather than the symptomatic and subjective feeling status of the patient.

12. Reference: Lewinsohn, P.M. and Clark, J.R. (1965) A factor analytically derived scale: For rating psychiatric patients in occupational therapy: Part II. Concurrent validity. AJOT, 19, 72-75.

D. 1. PRE-VOCATIONAL EVALUATION OF REHABILITATION POTENTIAL

2. Date Published: 1968

3. Author: David A. Ethridge, PhD, OTR

4. Citation: Ethridge. D.A. (1968) Pre-vocational assessment of rehabilitative potential of psychiatric patients. AJOT, 22, 161-167.

5. Target Population: The rating scale was developed by the author at Northville State Hospital in Michigan as a pilot project for psychiatric inpatients (70% were diagnosed as schizophrenic, 26% had some type of personality disorder, and the remaining 4% were diagnosed as psychoneurotic). A total of 421 evaluations were completed during a three-year pilot project. Of this total, 55% of the clients were female and 45% were male with an age range of 16 to 60 and a mean age of 32.4.

6. Variables Assessed: The rating scale is broken down into four major areas: work skills, habits, and tolerance; socialization, attitude toward others; personality characteristics; and general observation. Each of these four scales is further analyzed into specific skills related to potential for successful vocational placement. The rating scale is described in Appendix L.

7. Measurement Scales: The occupational therapist rates the patient on a 4-point scale (ordinal measurement) from very

poor performance (1 on the scale) to excellent (4 on the scale) for each of the 20 items.

8. Administration of Instrument: The rating scale is an observational instrument that is completed by the occupational therapist or work supervisor as in instances where the patient is engaged in a hospital work assignment. The rating scale can be used for specific time periods, such as one week, to measure progress in work adjustment, or over a longer period as a vehicle to assess potential for special placement in a sheltered workshop or community employment.

9. Scoring and Interpretation of Results: During the three-year pilot project in which 421 evaluations were completed, the mean score obtained on the scale was 61.1. The possible range of scores is 20 (very poor) and 80 (excellent) on the 20 items. The author states that a score of 60 or above indicates good work adjustment, while a score below 60 indicates relatively poor work adjustment.

10. Reliability and Validity Data: Reliability data are not reported. Further research is indicated to determine the reliability of the instrument. A question remains regarding the subjectivity of the ratings. For example, would occupational therapists rating the patient independently arrive at the same conclusions? The author reports that the instrument has good predictive validity. Out of 421 patients evaluated, 368 patients completed their rehabilitation programs successfully. The case records, from the State Division of Vocational Rehabilitation, were analyzed in compiling the outcome data.

11. Other Comments: The most important implication of this pre-vocational rating scale is "felt to be ...the factual information the coordinator gains by studying the individual item responses. Information regarding how each client relates to peers and authority, punctuality and attendance, sociability ...are important to the coordinator in developing the rehabilitation plan" (p. 161).

E. 1. COMPREHENSIVE EVALUATION OF BASIC LIVING SKILLS

2. Date Published: 1976
3. Authors: Jean Starr Casanova, OTR and Julie Ferber, OTR
4. Citation: Casanova, J.S. and Ferber, J. (1976) Comprehensive evaluation of basic living skills. AJOT, 30, 101-105.

5. Target Population: The evaluation scale was developed at Mendota Mental Health Institute in Madison, Wisconsin for chronic psychiatric inpatients.

6. Variables Assessed: The areas assessed include personal care and hygiene, housekeeping, meal planning and serving, use of telephone, bus transportation, functional reading and writing abilities, understanding of time, money use, and solving practical math problems.

7. Measurement Scales: The instrument is an observation checklist where the therapist rates on a 1-to-4 ordinal scale the client's behavior. The checklists are described in Appendices M and N.

8. Administration of Instrument: The Personal Care and Hygiene Checklist can be filled out very quickly by observing the client in the home or in a hospital. On the other hand, the occupational therapist observing the client using a bus, telephoning a store, or preparing a meal must be present while the client actually performs the activity. The written evaluation of reading and math abilities takes approximately one-half to one hour to administer.

9. Scoring and Interpretation of Results: At present, there are no norms for the instrument. The rating scale can be best used as an indication of individual client progress from the time of admission to discharge.

10. Reliability and Validity: No data are reported as to the reliability and validity of the instrument with psychiatric patients.

11. Other Comments: Further research is needed to determine the accuracy of using the instrument as a standardized rating scale. Norms, reliability and validity data would strengthen the use of the instrument in chronic psychiatric settings where the clients have lost basic ADL skills due to the nature of institutional living arrangements.

F. 1. THE INDEPENDENT LIVING SKILLS EVALUATION (ILSE)

2. Date Published: 1980

3. Authors: Toni Pan Johnson, OTR, Brenda Johanson-Vinnicombe, OTR, and Gary W. Merrill, AB

4. Citation: Johnson. T.P., Vinnicombe, B.J. and Merrill, G.W. (1980) The Independent Living Skills Evaluation. Occupational Therapy in Mental Health, 2, 5-18.

5. Target Population: The ILSE was developed in conjunction with an apartment-living program for chronic emotionally

disturbed individuals. The clients were between 18 and 64 years of age.

6. Variables Assessed: The ILSE is divided into 10 major categories:
   a) Money management (banking, budgeting, managing income)
   b) Shopping and consumer education
   c) Meal preparation and storage
   d) House cleaning and maintenance
   e) Personal hygiene and clothing maintenance
   f) Medication management and health care (self-care)
   g) Community resources and transportation
   h) Communication and interpersonal relations
   i) Problem-solving and decision-making
   j) Vocational and personal growth (time management, leisure skills)

7. Measurement Scales: Each of the 10 categories is subdivided into specific areas. Each of the subcategories were graded on a 1-to-4 ordinal scale, with 1 describing the lowest level of functioning, and 4 the optimal or highest level of functioning. Behavioral descriptions were developed for each subcategory scale.

8. Administration of Instrument: After the occupational therapist orients the client to the ILSE by explaining the purpose of the test and a description of the 10 areas evaluated, the client rates himself based on the written criteria. The evaluator also rates the client independently based on the evaluator's observations of the client's skill levels. The evaluator and clients then discuss each other's evaluation and a final score is determined. The authors report that the total evaluation takes about 2½ hours to complete. The evaluation is usually divided into three sessions.

9. Scoring and Interpretation of Results: The results of the ILSE are used to establish short-term and long-term treatment objectives for independent living that is formalized into a "learning contract" agreed upon by both the client and therapist. Clients are re-evaluated periodically and new treatment objectives are established.

10. Reliability and Validity Data: Reliability and validity data have not been reported. However, Marks,[17] in reviewing ILSE stated that "The validity of the ILSE is its ability to accurately assess an individual's ability to live independently" (p. 19).

Marks suggested that the authors administer the instrument to two independent groups—one clearly able to function independently and the other a dependent group. If the ISLE is indeed valid, the scores would significantly vary in the two groups.

11. Other Comments: The ILSE is a good model that occupational therapists can use in developing specific instruments linked to treatment programs. It is practical, easily administered and a good example of the potential value of occupational therapy in a community based treatment program.

12. Reference: Marks, R. (1980) Validating the ILSE, Occupational Therapy in Mental Health, 2, 19-20.

Summary

The analysis of assessment instruments published from 1961 to 1987 indicates that progress is being made to upgrade the practice of psychiatric occupational therapy. As these tests become more widely used in practice and research data are collected to establish normative samples, the tests will become more valuable in treatment planning, clinical research, and in quality assurance.

References

1. Hopkins HL and Smith HD (eds) (1983). Willard and Spackman's Occupational Therapy (6th ed). Philadelphia: Lippincott.

2. Sundberg N (1971). Assessment of Persons. Englewood Cliffs, New Jersey: Prentice-Hall.

3. Cynkin S (1979). Occupational Therapy: Toward Health Through Activities. Boston: Little, Brown and Co.

4. Glaser R (1963). Instructional technology and the measurement of learning outcomes. American Psychologist 18, 510-522.

5. Anastasi A (1982). Psychological Testing (5th ed). New York: Macmillan.

6. Casanova J and Ferber J (1976). Comprehensive evaluation of basic living skills. Am J Occup Ther 30, 101-105.

7. Johnson TP, Vinnicombe BJ, and Merrill GW (1980) The independent living skills evaluation. Occupational Therapy in Mental Health 2, 5-18.

8. Leonardelli C (in press). Milwaukee Evaluation of Daily Living Skills.

9. Maguire GH (1985). Activities of daily living, in Lewis C (ed): Aging: The Health Care Challenge. Philadelphia: Davis.

10. Moorhead L (1969). The occupational history. Am J Occup Ther 23, 329-334.
11. Florey LL and Michelman SM (1982). Occupational role history: A screening tool for psychiatric occupational therapy. Am J Occup Ther 36, 301-308.
12. Ethridge DA (1968). Pre-vocational assessment of rehabilitation potential of psychiatric patients Am J Occup Ther 22, 161-167.
13. American Psychiatric Association (1980). Diagnostic and Statistical Manual of Mental Disorders (3rd ed). Washington D.C.: American Psychiatric Association.
14. Clark J, Koch BA, and Nichols RC (1965). A factor analytically derived scale: For rating psychiatric patients in occupational therapy. Am J Occup Ther 19, 14-18.
15. Terman LM and Merrill MA (1960). Stanford-Binet Intelligence Scale: Manual for the Third Revision, Form L-M. Boston: Houghton Mifflin.
16. Schmidt RT and Toews JV (1970). Grip strength as measured by the Jamar dynamometer. Archives of Physical Medicine in Rehabilitation 51, 321-327.
17. Marks R (1980) Validating the I.L.S.E. Occupational Therapy in Mental Health 1, 19-20.
18. Buck JN (1948) The house-tree-person technique: A qualitative and quantitative scoring manual. J Clinical Psychology. (Monogram Supplement, Number 5).

APPENDICES

APPENDIX A
ROLE CHECKLIST

NAME _____ AGE _____ DATE _____

SEX: ☐ MALE   ☐ FEMALE   ARE YOU RETIRED: ☐ YES   ☐ NO

MARITAL STATUS:

☐ SINGLE   ☐ MARRIED   ☐ SEPARATED   ☐ DIVORCED   ☐ WIDOWED

The purpose of this checklist is to identify the major roles in your life. The checklist, which is divided into two parts, presents 10 roles and defines each one.

PART I

Beside each role, indicate, by checking the appropriate column, if you performed the role in the past, if you presently perform the role, and if you plan to perform the role in the future. You may check more than one column for each role. For example, if you volunteered in the past, do not volunteer at present, but plan to in the future, you would check the past and future columns.

ROLE	PAST	PRESENT	FUTURE
STUDENT: Attending school on a part-time or full-time basis.			
WORKER: Part-time or full-time paid employment.			
VOLUNTEER: Donating services, *at least once a week,* to a hospital, school, community, political campaign, and so forth.			
CARE GIVER: Responsibility, *at least once a week,* for the care of someone such as a child, spouse, relative, or friend.			
HOME MAINTAINER: Responsibility, *at least once a week,* for the upkeep of the home such as housecleaning or yardwork.			

APPENDIX A

PART I *(continued)*

FRIEND: Spending time or doing something, *at least once a week,* with a friend.			
FAMILY MEMBER: Spending time or doing something, *at least once a week,* with a family member such as a child, spouse, parent, or other relative.			
RELIGIOUS PARTICIPANT: Involvement, *at least once a week,* in groups or activities affiliated with one's religion (excluding worship).			
HOBBYIST/AMATEUR: Involvement, *at least once a week,* in a hobby or amateur activity such as sewing, playing a musical instrument, woodworking, sports, the theater, or participation in a club or team.			
PARTICIPANT IN ORGANIZATIONS: Involvement, *at least once a week,* in organizations such as the American Legion, National Organization for Women, Parents Without Partners, Weight Watchers, and so forth.			
OTHER: _____ A role not listed which you have performed, are presently performing, and/or plan to perform. Write the role on the line above and check the appropriate column(s).			

Reprinted by permission of the author, Frances Oakley, MS, OTR.

APPENDIX B
ROLE CHECKLIST

PART II

The same roles are listed below. Next to *each* role, check the column which best indicates how valuable or important the role is to you. Answer for *each* role, even if you have never performed or do not plan to perform the role.

ROLE	NOT AT ALL VALUABLE	SOME-WHAT VALUABLE	VERY VALUABLE
STUDENT: Attending school on a part-time or full-time basis.			
WORKER: Part-time or full-time paid employment.			
VOLUNTEER: Donating services, *at least once a week,* to a hospital, school, community, political campaign, and so forth.			
CARE GIVER: Responsibility, *at least once a week,* for the care of someone such as a child, spouse, relative, or friend.			
HOME MAINTAINER: Responsibility, *at least once a week,* for the upkeep of the home such as housecleaning or yardwork.			
FRIEND: Spending time or doing something, *at least once a week,* with a friend.			

APPENDIX B

PART II *(continued)*

FAMILY MEMBER: Spending time or doing something, *at least once a week,* with a family member such as a child, spouse, parent, or other relative.			
RELIGIOUS PARTICIPANT: Involvement, *at least once a week,* in groups or activities affiliated with one's religion (excluding worship).			
HOBBYIST/AMATEUR: Involvement, *at least once a week,* in a hobby or amateur activity such as sewing, playing a musical instrument, woodworking, sports, the theater, or participation in a club or team.			
PARTICIPANT IN ORGANIZATIONS: Involvement, *at least once a week,* in organizations such as the American Legion, National Organization for Women, Parents Withour Partners, Weight Watchers, and so forth.			
OTHER:_____ A role not listed which you have performed, are presently performing, and/ or plan to perform. Write the role on the line above and check the appropriate column(s).			

APPENDIX C

NPI INTEREST CHECKLIST

Name: _____ Unit: _____ Date: _____

Please check each item below according to your interest.

INTEREST

ACTIVITY	CASUAL	STRONG	NO
1. Gardening			
2. Sewing			
3. Poker			
4. Languages			
5. Social Clubs			
6. Radio			
7. Bridge			
8. Car Repair			
9. Writing			
10. Dancing			
11. Needlework			
12. Golf			
13. Football			
14. Popular Music			
15. Puzzles			
16. Holidays			
17. Solitaire			
18. Movies			
19. Lectures			
20. Swimming			
21. Bowling			
22. Visiting			
23. Mending			
24. Chess			
25. Barbecues			
26. Reading			
27. Traveling			
28. Manual Arts			
29. Parties			
30. Dramatics			
31. Shuffleboard			
32. Ironing			
33. Social Studies			
34. Classical Music			
35. Floor Mopping			
36. Model Building			
37. Baseball			
38. Checkers			
39. Singing			
40. Home Repairs			

APPENDIX C
NPI INTEREST CHECKLIST

INTEREST

ACTIVITY	CASUAL	STRONG	NO

41. Exercise
42. Volleyball
43. Woodworking
44. Billiards
45. Driving
46. Dusting
47. Jewelry Making
48. Tennis
49. Cooking
50. Basketball

51. History
52. Guitar
53. Science
54. Collecting
55. Ping Pong
56. Leatherwork
57. Shopping
58. Photography
59. Painting
60. Television

61. Concerts
62. Ceramics
63. Camping
64. Laundry
65. Dating
66. Mosaics
67. Politics
68. Scrabble
69. Decorating
70. Math

71. Service Groups
72. Piano
73. Scouting
74. Plays
75. Clothes
76. Knitting
77. Hairstyling
78. Religion
79. Drums
80. Conversation

Please list other special interests:

Matsutsuyn J., The NPI Interest Check List, *AJOT 23* (4), 1969.
Reprinted with permission from the American Occupational Therapy Association.

APPENDIX D
MILWAUKEE EVALUATION OF DAILY LIVING SKILLS (MEDLS)
Screening Form

Client _____ Date _____

Age _____ Sex _____ No. _____ Evaluator _____

		Skill Area	Status*	**Not known at this time
I.		Basic Communication Skills		
II.		Eating		
IV.		Maintenance of clothing		
V.		Medication Management		
VI.	A.	Toileting		
VI.	B.	Brushing Teeth		
VI.	C.	Denture Care		
VI.	D.	Bathing		
VI.	E.	Use of Make-up		
VI.	F.	Shaving		
VI.	G.	Nail Care		
VI.	H.	Hair Care		
VI.	I.	Eyeglass Care		
VII.		Personal Health Care		
VIII.		Safety in Community		
IX.		Safety in Home		
X.		Time Awareness		
XI.		Use of Money		
XII.		Use of Telephone		
XIII.		Use of Transportation		

* Based on evaluator's review of the medical record, information from others, initial observations and/or itial interview, use the following key:

    I = independent in this skill area

    E = evaluation needed in this skill area

    NA = not applicable to client (e.g. due to gender, physical or behavioral limitation, etc.)

** "Not known at this time" is marked when evaluator does not have enough information on which to decide if client is "independent" or "evaluation needed." *This item should be rechecked* when evaluator is more familiar with client.

APPENDIX E
Milwaukee Evaluation of Daily Living Skills
Sample Subtest

7. Eyeglass Care
Method: Performance of skills
Equipment:
glasses
kleenex
Procedure: Instruct the client:
"Please clean your glasses and show me how you store them when you are not wearing them."
Ask the client:
   "What would you do if your glasses were broken?"

Skill List:	**Key Words**
a. Cleans glasses	cleans
b. Stores glasses safely	storage
c. states: call or go to the eye doctor	repair
take to the eyeglass clinic or store	
fix myself (if minor repair)	

Maximum time: 3 minutes
Scoring:
3 = Performs all skills
2 = Performs 2 of 3 skills (list *one* deficit using key words)
1 = Performs 1 of 3 skills (list *two* deficit using key word)
0 = Unable to perform any skills

APPENDIX F

Milwaukee Evaluation of Daily Living Skills (MEDLS)
Reporting Form

Patient _____ Sex _____ No. _____ Date _____ Evaluator _____

Skill Area	Maximum Points Possible	Score Attained or NEN*	Key Words	Re-test date Score Attained or NEN*	Key Words
I. Basic Communication Skills	4				
II. Dressing	4/2				
III. Eating	6				
IV. Maintenance of clothing	4				
V. Medication Management	6/5				
VI. A. Toileting	3/5				
IV. B. Brushing Teeth	4				
VI. C. Denture Care	4				
VI. D. Bathing	3				
VI. E. Use of Make-Up	2				
VI. F. Shaving	4				

APPENDIX F *(continued)*

Skill Area	Maximum Points Possible	Score Attained or NEN*	Key Words	Re-test date Score Attained or NEN*	Key Words
VI. G. Nail Care	4				
VI. H. Hair Care	3				
VI. I. Eyeglass Care	3				
VII. Personal Health Care	4				
VIII. Safety in Community	4				
IX. Safety in Home	3/3				
X. Time Awareness	6				
XI. Use of Money	3				
XII. Use of Telephone	4				
XIII. Use of Transportation	5				

* NEN - No Evaluation Needed
  Comment:

Evaluator's signature _____
Evaluator's signature (re-test) _____

APPENDIX G

MFRS. REHAB. RATING SCALE

Patient's name _____ Rater's name _____ Date _____

RESPONSE TO WORK, ACTIVITY OR TASK

I.	Interest in work, activity or task:	little or none	_____	considerable
II.	Ability to initiate work or activity:	little or none	_____	considerable
III.	Ability to follow through with a job:	little or none	_____	considerable
IV.	Ability to take direction:	little or none	_____	considerable
V.	Ability to work with others:	little or none	_____	considerable
VI.	Quality of work (how good the work is):	poor	_____	good
VII.	Quantity of work (how much work is done):	little or none	_____	considerable

RESPONSE TO PEOPLE (socialization)

VIII.	Attitude toward fellow patients:	indifferent	_____	friendly
IX.	Observed hostility:	extreme	_____	little or none
X.	Quantity of verbalization (how much patient talks):			
	A. not at all			
	B. talks continuously			
XI.	Content of verbalization (how well patient talks):	"gibberish"	_____	normal
XII.	Participation in social activities:	little or none	_____	sensible, enthusiastic

GENERAL OBSERVATIONS

XIII.	Independence (how well patient seems able to take care of self:	not at all	_____	adequately
XIV.	Dependability:	unpredictable	_____	dependable
XV.	General conduct:	inappropriate	_____	appropriate

COMMENTS

From Wolf, R.J. (1961). A behavior rating scale. *AJOT*, 15, p.14. Reprinted with permission.

APPENDIX H

Minnesota Follow-Up Study Rehabilitation Rating Scale (MFRS)
Instructions for Filling Out The Rating Scale

Below you will find 15 different scales, each one showing one way in which a person can be observed. Each scale runs from one extreme to the other, from "bad" to "good," from "abnormal" to "normal." Please indicate by placing a check mark (X) in the right place, indicating where you would rate the person you are observing on that particular scale.

Look at each scale separately. Do not try to give an overall impression since people differ not only in the overall impression they create, but especially in how they appear in these different areas: for instance, a patient might be a good worker, but he does not talk at all, or a patient might get along very well with other patients in a group activity, but is unable to do work.

It will not always be possible to choose one spot on the scale that fits a particular person best; do not check more than one place on any one scale.

As you will notice, only the extreme positions on scales are described. All five positions should be equally considered; however, before you make a rating, it will help if you read the descriptions. Try to get an idea of what you should judge on each scale. If you get a feeling for what the scale as a whole describes, you will be able to fill in for yourself what the other three boxes mean.

If the patient's behavior has changed since you last rated him, please rate only as he is now, today—do not try to judge "average" behavior.

From Wolf R.J. (1981) A behavior rating scale. *AJOT.* 15, p 14. Reprinted with permission.

APPENDIX I
Diagnostic Occupational Therapy Test Protocol

Patient's Name:
Patient's Number:
Ward:
Doctor:
Date:
General Observations: (Include neatness, facial expression, posture, gait, any mannerism, initial attitude toward therapist and test):

House*
Will you please draw a house?
1. Where is the house located?
2. Whose house were you thinking about while you were drawing?
3. What kind of people live in that house?

Tree
Will you please draw a tree?
1. What kind of a tree is that?
2. Is the tree living or dead?
3. What does that tree make you think of?
4. What is the weather like?

Person*
Will you please draw a person?
1. Who is the person?
2. What is the person doing?
3. How does the person feel?
4. How old is the person?

Painting
MATERIALS:
A sheet of 8½" × 11" white paper, 2 or 3 different sizes and a set of Prang water colors (8 colors).
TIME:
1. Tell me about your painting.
2. Why did you use those colors?
COMMENTS:

Leather
MATERIALS:
Two 2½" × 1¾" squares of tooling leather.
Water and sponge
Five designs of lettering
Four background designs
Pencil
Tracing paper
Swivel cutter
No. 1 beveling tool
Backgrounder*
Pearshader*
Veiner*
Flowertool*
DIRECTIONS:
Show patient samples of lettering and ask him to choose one of each to reproduce on leather. Instruct him in method of transforming initials and background onto leather and carving it.
TIME:
COMMENTS:

APPENDIX I *(continued)*

Ceramics

DIRECTIONS: Give patient a 10″ ball of clay on a large bat and a dish of water and ask him to make something.

TIME:

QUESTIONS:
1. Tell me about what you have made.

COMMENTS: (Include method of working clay aggressiveness. How much clay used, attitude toward clay, how much water used, comments made).

---

*Questions taken from Buck's The House-Tree-Person Test.[18]

Checkerboard

DIRECTIONS:
Give patient the empty checkerboard and wooden pieces. Tell him it is a checkerboard and ask him to arrange it.

TIME:

ORDER OF ARRANGEMENT:

COMMENTS (Methods, mannerisms, comments by the patient): If patient comments upon missing squares, ask him, "What do you think you should do about it?"

TIME:

DIAGRAM:

COMMENTS:

---

*Manufactured by Craftool.

From Clark I.R., et al. (1965). A factor analytically derived scale for rating psychiatric patients in occupational therapy. *AJOT,* 19, p. 17-18. Reprinted with permission.

APPENDIX J

Occupational Therapy Trait Rating Scale (OTTRS)
Administration

Instructions to Raters: Rate only those patients whom you know well. A two-week period of observation is a suggested minimum. Circle the number on a scale which represents the behavior most typical of a patient. Make only one rating per item. Do not hesitate to make ratings on the extreme ends of scales when appropriate. A U to be circled when a behavior has not been observed is provided at the right of each item. However, use the unobserved column as infrequently as possible.

Scoring Procedure: This scale yields five separate scores corresponding to the factors derived in the original study. To obtain the score for each factor or dimension, simply sum the ratings which a patient receives on the items included within the dimension. The five dimensions and the items subsumed under them following: I. Creativity. Items 1, 2, 3.

II. Dominance-Manipulativeness. Items 4, 5, 6, 7.

III. Energy-Enthusiasm. Items 8, 9, 10, 11.

IV. Social Isolation. Items 12, 13, 14, 15, 16.

V. Orderliness. Items 17, 18, 19, 20, 21.

From Clark, I.R., et al. (1965). A factor analytically derived scale for rating psychiatric patients in occupational therapy. *AJOT,* 19. p 17-18. Reprinted with permission.

APPENDIX K

OCCUPATIONAL THERAPY TRAIT RATING SCALE

Patient's Name _____   Rater _____   Date _____

1. How much creativity does patient show in his use of materials?

1	2	3		U
none-ordinary use of materials	somewhat creative	very creative		

2. Amount of group influence.

1	2	3		U
shows group influence in choice of project	shows some influence, but integrates this with own ideas	wants to make something entirely different from others		

3. How utilitarian is the patient's usual project?

1	2	3		U
chooses to make utilitarian object with no unnecessary embellishments	chooses to make utilitarian objects but with an artistic flair	chooses to make something artistic		

4. How much does the patient dominate or seek to dominate personnel?

1	2	3	4	5	U
never	sometimes	frequently	almost always		

5. How much does the patient dominate or seek to dominate other patients?

1	2	3	4	5	U
never	sometimes	frequently	almost always		

6. How often does the patient try to Manipulate Personnel (e.g., to get special favors, attention, materials, therapist to do work for him, etc.)

1	2	3	4	5	U
never	occasionally	frequently	very frequently		

7. How much fluctuation does patient show in mood, interest, and performance?

1	2	3	4	5	U
none	mild	moderate	extreme		

APPENDIX K *(continued)*

Patient's Name _____ **Rater** _____ **Date** _____

8. How much energy does the patient put forth in his work?

1	2	3	4	5	U
minimal to the point of insufficiency to successfully complete project	keeps working but conservative energy	uses average amount of energy	"works up a sweat"	excessive to the point of fatigue	

9. How much enthusiasm does patient usually show in projects?

1	2	3	4	5	U
seems to be completely lacking in interest	not too interested	average amount of interest	tend to be enthusiastic	seems to be extremely enthusiastic over project	

10. At what speed does patient work?

1	2	3	4	5	U
works so slowly that almost at a standstill	works slowly	average rate of speed	works fast	works at extremely accelerated speed	

11. In what manner does patient usually approach activities?

1	2	3	4	5	U
unusually passive, e.g., barely taps material when pounding metal bowl	somewhat passive	uses appropriate approach for media used	somewhat aggressive	unusually aggressive for media being used, e.g., tries to bludgeon nail into board with one blow. "Whacks" cloth	

12. What is the degree of the patient's association with others?

1	2	3	4	5	U
almost always in the company of others	often in the company of others	about equally alone and with others	usually by himself, mixes sometimes	always stays by himself, ignores everyone	

APPENDIX K *(continued)*

Patient's Name   Rater   Date

13. How well liked does patient seem to be?

1	2	3	4	5	U
patient seems very well liked by other patients, is sought out by them, is center of group	patient seems moderately well liked by others	others appear to be neutral toward patient	patient seems somewhat liked	patient appears quite unpopular, may be actively disparaged or ignored by others	

14. How active is the patient in seeking contact with the same sex? (think of activity in terms of seeking out members of the same sex during coffee breaks, leaving work to associate with, etc.)

1	2	3	4	U
extremely active	moderately active in seeking contact	appears indifferent	appears to avoid contact	

15. How much help does the patient give others?

1	2	3	4	U
extremely helpful	somewhat helpful	rarely helpful	no help	

16. How active is the patient in seeking contact with the opposite sex? (think of activity in terms of seeking out members of the same sex during coffee breaks, leaving work to associate with, etc.)

1	2	3	4	U
extremely active	moderately active in seeking contact	appears indifferent to opposite sex	appears to avoid contact	

APPENDIX K *(continued)*

Patient's Name _____ Rater _____ Date _____

17. How much material does patient use?

1	2	3	4	5	U
very wasteful	somewhat wasteful	average	somewhat conservative	very conservative	

18. To what degree is patient able to plan ahead and work in an orderly fashion?

1	2	3	4	5	U
shows no ability; haphazards in work	tends to be poorly organized	fairly well organized	shows a high degree of organization in work		

19. At what degree of precision does the patient work?

1	2	3	4	5	U
no concern for detail, works in sloppy manner	some tendency to be careless	average degree of precision	works very neatly	overly meticulous with unusual concern for detail	

20. Does patient abuse tools or equipment used in occupational therapy?

1	2	3	U
frequently	occasionally	never	

21. What is the amount of bizarreness entering into patient's productions?

1	2	3	4	U
exceedingly bizarre	moderately bizarre	borderline, productions somewhat peculiar	no bizarreness	

From Clark, J.R. et al. (1965). A factor analytically derived scale for rating psychiatric patients in occupational therapy. *AJOT, 19,* pp. 17-18. Reprinted with permission.

APPENDIX L
Pre-Vocational Evaluation of Rehabilitation Potential

NAME _____

DATE _____

RATER _____

ASSIGNMENT _____

WORK SKILLS, HABITS AND TOLERANCE

1. Interest, motivation or enthusiasm	Little or none, Indifferent	Poor, Ambivalent Slow to interest	Acceptable Fair	Eager, absorbed Good or excellent
2. Initiative, ability to initiate activity, energy output	Little or none, Can't start job	Poor, slow to get started	Adequate, applies self to job	Energetic, initiates jobs, absorbed
3. Ability to follow through, concentration, attention span	Little or none, Distractible	Poor, needs reminding	Adequate attention, Satisfactory	Attention good, Hard to mislead
4. Ability to take directions or authority accepting of suggestions, response to controls	Poor, resentful, hostile, critical, Resents authority	Avoiding, openly defiant Debates suggestions	Accepting, tolerant, Responds to suggestions	Good, adequate, Responds well
5. Quality of workmanship, neatness, accuracy, manual dexterity	Inept, careless, slovenly	Poor, below average Untidy, errors	Passable, acceptable Improving skills	Neat, exact, few mistakes, adequate
6. Quantity of work, production	Little or none, Unacceptable	Below standards, Less than required	Average or acceptable, spasmodic	Good, above average, Considerable work
7. Attendance, punctuality, regularity	Irregular, late, habitual absence	Unpredictable, often late, inconsistent	Usually prompt, Fairly consistent	Regular, puntual, Stays overtime

APPENDIX L *(continued)*

SOCIALIZATION, ATTITUDE TOWARD OTHERS

1. Participation in social activities	Never participant, Stays to himself	Occasionally attends, Little participation	Goes regularly, some participation	Enjoys activities, Active participant
2. Verbalization, quantity and content	Talks, constantly, confused, rambling OR Doesn't talk	Chatters, often rambling OR Underproductive	Responds to conversation, No unusual speech	Appropriate, enjoys conversation Initiates discussions
3. Aggressivity, hostility	Extremely high, Irritates others	Sometimes causes problems	Occasional but no problems	None noticed, Appropriate
4. Thoughtfulness, peer adjustment	Belittles others, Non-sharing, taker	Doesn't share, indifferent	Notices others and needs, shares	Praises properly, Interested in others
5. Ability to work with others, cooperativeness	Unable to adjust, Hostile, withdrawn Antagonizes others	Stubborn, distant Aloof, critical, Irritable	Quiet, but friendly, Generally acceptable, fits in	Stimulates others, Active, friendly, Group participant

APPENDIX L *(continued)*

PERSONALITY CHARACTERISTICS

1. Unusual behavior or mannerisms	Hallucinates, gestures, bizarre	Occasionally noted, Can be controlled	Rare inappropriate behavior	Actions never unusual
2. Anxiety	Extremely high, Easily produced OR Extremely low, Apathetic	Sensitive, often observed, Interfers with work	Moderately anxious, sometimes affects work	Casual, normal and appropriate
3. Judgement, dependability, responsibility	Irresponsible, inaccurate, oversteps authority	Needs reminding, Often inaccurate, Not dependable	Average, accepts responsibility, Usually reliable	Sound in judgment, Eager to advance
4. Frustration tolerance, self-control, emotional control	Verbal abuse, destructive, temper tantrums	Occasional poor control, moody	Mood seldom affects work, shows self-control	Very stable, well controlled

APPENDIX L *(continued)*

GENERAL OBSERVATIONS

1. Appearance	Slovenly, unkempt Inappropriate	Occasionally sloppy careless	Acceptable, Usually presentable	Appropriate, well-groomed
2. Learning capacity, general intelligence	Slow or faulty, Unable to learn	Slow to catch on, poor retention	Able to learn with instruction	Learns rapidly, Remembers well
3. Knowledge of equipment, safety and shop policies	Needs help constantly, forgets procedures, hazard	Partial knowledge, Some mistakes, a few accidents	Learn correct procedures, a safe worker	Can repair requipment, safe, protects others
4. Use of time	Dawdles, can't make up mind, Unorganized	Wastes time, poor organization, Slow at decisions	Usually on the job, Manages situations	Efficient, always busy, accurate and fast

ADDITIONAL COMMENTS:

From Ethridge, D.A. (1968). Pre-vocational assessment of rehabilitative potential of psychiatric patients. *AJOT*, 22. p 163. Reprinted with permission.

APPENDIX M
Comprehensive Evaluation of Basic Living Skills
CHECK LIST FOR PRACTICAL EVALUATION

NAME _____

CLIENT NO _____

SCORE _____

RATING

Observe the client performing the following skills. Place the number corresponding to the client's correct level of function in the blank preceding each skill.

     4. Performs skill independently and correctly.

     3. Requires some assistance to perform skill correctly.

     2. Requires much assistance to perform skill correctly.

     1. Cannot perform skill independently.

Indicate N/A if the item is not applicable.

PART ONE: Meal Planning

____ knowledge of basic four

____ menu planning

____ formation of grocery list

____ handle milk carton

PART TWO: Telephone

____ use of telephone book

____ depositing dime

____ dialing

____ asking information

____ use appropriate social behavior on phone ("hello," "thank you," etc.)

____ retaining information

PART THREE: Bus

____ what bus to take

____ location of bus stop

____ distance from bus stops to hospital and store

____ times bus arrives at bus stops

____ time it takes to walk to bus stop

____ how to board bus

____ how much money bus costs

____ where to stand at stop

____ how to tell which bus to get on

____ how long to stay on the bus

____ where to get off

____ how to inform bus driver to stop

____ how much time it takes to get to store, do shopping and get back

____ how much time at disposal

____ what bus to take back

PART FOUR: Shopping

____ comparative shopping

____ look for quality in fruits, vegetables, etc.

____ pay clerk

____ check change

____ put things away in proper place

PART FIVE: Meal Preparation

____ can follow recipe

____ get things from refrigerator

____ get utensils and pans from cupboard

____ break eggs

____ operate small appliances (toaster, electric mixer, etc.)

____ adequate stirring techniques

____ peel, cut, fruits/vegetables

____ can prepare fried foods

____ can prepare baked foods

____ can prepare boiled foods

APPENDIX M *(continued)*

PART SIX: Serving and Eating
___ serve food appropriately
___ offer food to others
___ pass food at table
___ appropriate use of napkin
___ maintain suitable posture
___ appropriate use of utensils
___ drinking from cup or glass
___ pour from pitcher
___ adequate chewing motions

PART SEVEN: Meal Clean-Up
___ clear table
___ put away food
___ scrape and stack dishes
___ wash dishes
___ wash pots and pans
___ wipe off work areas, table
___ dry dishes
___ put dishes, pans, utensils, in proper
    storage areas
___ remove dishwater
___ clean dish cloth and sink
___ sweep floor

SCORING
sum of ratings: _____
number of N/A items × four: _____
Practical Evaluation Score:

List any additional skills the client has difficulty performing:

signature   Title
administered by
_____
Signature   Title
_____
date

From Casanova, J.S. and Ferber, J. (1976). Comprehensive evaluation of basic
living skills. *AJOT,* 30. p 102. Reprinted with permission.

APPENDIX N
Comprehensive Evaluation of Basic Living Skills (continued)
CHECK LIST FOR PERSONAL CARE AND HYGIENE
NAME _____
CLIENT NO _____
SCORE _____

RATING

Observe the client performing the following skills. Place the number corresponding to the client's correct level of function in the blank preceding each skill.

4. Performs skill independently and correctly.

3. Requires some assistance to perform skill correctly.

2. Requires much assistance to perform skill correctly.

1. Cannot perform skill independently or correctly.

Indicate N/A if the item is not applicable.

Toileting

___ control of bowel and bladder needs

___ get on toilet

___ adjust clothing

___ use of toilet paper

___ get off toilet

___ re-adjust clothing

___ flush toilet

Brushing Teeth

___ put toothpaste on brush

___ proper brushing motions

___ rinse mouth

Bathing

___ operate faucets in sink

___ operate faucets in tub or shower

___ adequate use of soap

___ adequate use of towel, wash cloth

___ able to get in and out of bathtub or shower

___ wash hands

___ wash face

Hair Care

___ shampoo hair

___ dry hair

___ set hair

___ comb and brush hair in organized way

Dressing

___ choose adequate clothing appropriate for physical/social situation

___ put on undergarments

___ put on shirts, blouses

___ put on pants or dress

___ operate fasteners

___ put on and lace, tie shoes

___ put on and buckle belt

___ hang up clothing

___ put on coat, hat, scarf, gloves

___ glasses (clean, put back in case)

APPENDIX N *(continued)*

Make-Up
___ apply base, powder, lipstick, eye make-up
___ use proper amount when applying

Shaving
___ adequate use of electric or safety razor
___ use razor safely

Posture
___ sit properly
___ walk appropriately

Nail Care
___ trim fingernails safely and neatly
___ trim toenails safely and neatly

Housekeeping
___ make a bed
___ dust
___ sweep/vacuum
___ launder clothes
___ iron clothes

SCORING

sum or ratings _____
number of N/A items × four _____
Personal Care and Hygiene Score _____

List any additional skills the client has difficulty performing.

administered by

_____

signature   Title

_____

date

Practical Evaluation Score:

From Casanova, J.S. and Ferber, J. (1976). Comprehensive evaluation of basic living skills. *AJOT,* 30. p. 104. Reprinted with permission.

INDEX

Page numbers in *in italic* refer to tables; page numbers **in boldface** refer to appendices